T0332358

Ashwagandha for Quality of Life

This book offers a comprehensive overview of the scientific evidence supporting the diverse health benefits of Ashwagandha. Each chapter delves into specific aspects, exploring its effects on stress management, cognitive function, physical performance, immune system support, sleep quality, and hormonal balance. Through an evidence-based approach, the text aims to bridge the gap between traditional wisdom and modern scientific understanding, presenting Ashwagandha as a promising herb for enhancing quality of life. *Ashwagandha for Quality of Life: Scientific Evidence* begins by highlighting the origin and botanical characteristics of Ashwagandha and explores the wide range of its traditional and modern applications. By identifying the main active compounds and their functions, readers gain insight into the herb's potential physiological effects. Further, the book investigates Ashwagandha's potential for preventing and treating COVID-19. The book is intended for the general readership, herbalists, naturopaths, alternative medicine practitioners, and life science/medical students and researchers to gain a comprehensive understanding of Ashwagandha's potential in improving health and well-being, while also emphasizing the importance of quality and chemotyping for optimal benefits.

Sustainable Industrial and Environmental Bioprocesses
Series Editor: Dr Ashok Pandey

This book series aims to provide a comprehensive collection of books focusing on bioprocesses in industrial and environmental biotechnology. The multidisciplinary content encompasses the chemical and biochemical engineering, industrial microbiology, and energy biosciences, all with a central theme of sustainable development and circular economy principles. The books align with the Sustainable Development Goals (SDGs) and offer state-of-the-art information and in-depth knowledge on the subject matter. The books in this series also emphasize on the application of emerging tools, such as machine learning and artificial intelligence, for the advancement of bioprocesses. While primarily targeting academicians and researchers, the series is valuable for policy planners and industry professionals, with carefully tailored contents to cater to their specific needs and interests.

Professor Ashok Pandey *is currently Distinguished Scientist at the Centre for Innovation and Translational Research, CSIR-Indian Institute of Toxicology Research, Lucknow, India. His major research and technological development interests are industrial & environmental biotechnology and energy biosciences, focusing on biomass to biofuels & chemicals, waste to wealth & energy, etc. He has 16 patents, 120 books, >1000 papers and book chapters, etc with h index of 131 and >74,000 citations. Professor Pandey is the recipient of many national and international awards and honours, which include Fellow, The World Academy of Sciences (TWAS), Highly Cited Researcher (Top 1% in the world), Clarivate Analytics (since 2018- till date), Rank #1 in India in Biology in India and Biochemistry and #417 in the world, Research.Com (2023), Rank #1 in India in Microbiology under Enabling and Strategic Technologies sector, Elsevier (2021), Rank #1 in India in Biotechnology and #8 in the world, Stanford University Report (2020-2021-2022), etc.*

Decentralized Sanitation and Water Treatment: Treatment in Cold Environments and Techno-Economic Aspects
R.D. Tyagi, Ashok Pandey, Patrick Drogui, Bhoomika Yadav, Sridhar Pilli and Jonathan W.C. Wong

Biodegradation of Toxic and Hazardous Chemicals: Detection and Mineralization
Kashyap K. Dubey, Kamal. K. Pant, Ashok Pandey and Maria Angeles Sanromán

Biodegradation of Toxic and Hazardous Chemicals: Remediation and Resource Recovery
Kashyap K. Dubey, Kamal K. Pant, Ashok Pandey and Maria Angeles Sanromán

Waste Management in Climate Change and Sustainability- Lignocellulosic Waste
Sunita Varjani, Izharul Haq, Ashok Pandey, Vijai Kumar Gupta, and Xuan-Thanh Bui

Ashwagandha for Quality of Life: Scientific Evidence
Sunil Kaul and Renu Wadhwa

Ashwagandha for Quality of Life
Scientific Evidence

Sunil Kaul and Renu Wadhwa

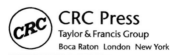

CRC Press
Taylor & Francis Group
Boca Raton London New York

CRC Press is an imprint of the
Taylor & Francis Group, an **informa** business

Designed cover image: Sunil Kaul and Renu Wadhwa

First edition published 2025
by CRC Press
2385 NW Executive Center Drive, Suite 320, Boca Raton FL 33431

and by CRC Press
4 Park Square, Milton Park, Abingdon, Oxon, OX14 4RN

CRC Press is an imprint of Taylor & Francis Group, LLC

© 2025 Sunil Kaul and Renu Wadhwa

ISBN: 9781032705675 (hbk)
ISBN: 9781032705729 (pbk)
ISBN: 9781032705743 (ebk)

DOI: 10.1201/9781032705743

Typeset in Times
by codeMantra

Contents

Foreword

In the pursuit of holistic well-being, mankind has sought nature's remedies since time immemorial. However, numerous herbs are enumerated for their beneficial potential, but few herbs have woven themselves as intricately into the fabric of healing as Ashwagandha. Scientifically known as *Withania somnifera*, this revered herb deeply rooted in Ayurveda emerges as a remarkable chapter in our age-old quest for optimal health. Its use in traditional Ayurvedic medicine spans centuries, with practitioners hailing its efficacy in promoting vitality, longevity, and overall well-being. Thus Ashwagandha has earned a distinguished reputation for its adaptogenic properties, supporting the body's ability to manage stress and maintain balance.

I am delighted to introduce the book *Ashwagandha for Quality of Life: Scientific Evidence*. This book delves into the fascinating world of Ashwagandha, exploring its origins, historical significance, molecular composition, and the wealth of therapeutic potential it harbors. The book is designed to help us understand not only what Ashwagandha is, but, more importantly, what it possesses — the medicinal treasures hidden within. The book has been meticulously structured to present every aspect of Ashwagandha in a systematic way, from traditional claims and active ingredients to modus operandi and up-to-date research.

Scientific validity is a cornerstone of understanding the true potential of any medicinal herb. This book meticulously examines the body of research that supports the traditional claims surrounding Ashwagandha. From controlled experiments to clinical trials, the evidence presented here forms a compelling narrative that bridges ancient wisdom with modern scientific rigor.

Intriguingly, the exploration extends to Ashwagandha's potential role in the realm of cancer prevention and treatment. This chapter in the book scrutinizes the anticancer ingredients and unravels the mechanisms through which they exhibit their therapeutic prowess, shedding light on promising avenues for future research.

As the world grapples with the unprecedented challenges posed by the COVID-19 pandemic, the book also addresses a question on many minds: Can Ashwagandha prevent and treat COVID-19? Through available evidence, this chapter explores the herb's potential role in supporting immune function and overall resilience.

The journey doesn't end here. The book contemplates the "what next" for Ashwagandha, considering emerging research, innovative applications, and the evolving landscape of integrative medicine. It provides a roadmap for those intrigued by the intricate chemistry of this botanical marvel.

Furthermore, the book offers a curated list of suggested readings, inviting readers to deepen their knowledge and understanding of Ashwagandha's diverse facets. This book stands as a testament to the enduring relevance of ancient wisdom in our quest for health and vitality.

I congratulate the authors; may this journey through the realms of Ashwagandha ignite curiosity, inspire contemplation, and empower readers with the knowledge to navigate the fascinating world of Ashwagandha.

With best wishes,
Prof. Tanuja Manoj Nesari
Director
All India Institute of Ayurveda (AIIA)
New Delhi

Preface

Quality of life has undergone significant changes over the past century. Advances in health care, quality of life, and standards of living have increased life expectancy and rapidly expanded the world's elderly population. Complicated social organization has led to changes in social and psychological health. Birth rates have declined. Industrialized lifestyles, including excessive use of chemicals, have contributed to increased stress and anxiety. Maintaining quality of life, especially by extending life expectancy, has become a new challenge in the current technological age.

Quality of life depends on many factors, including standard of living, hygiene, nutrition, environmental conditions, diseases, and therapeutics. It is extremely difficult to define the parameters for quality of life. While health is often thought of as a disease-free state, what is the exact cutoff that defines us as healthy or unhealthy? Are regular daily rhythms — such as waking up on time, feeling hungry, eating well, working regularly, and sleeping — signs of good health? We all have so much variation in these factors that it would be impossible to define good health by such specific measures. It is perhaps similar to a very spicy food that one person may enjoy, while another may have tears and an allergic reaction to. Unlike the man-made world, where uniformity and reproducibility are hallmarks of quality, biological systems are diverse and unique. No one set of parameters defines us as healthy or unhealthy, just as no one drug works perfectly for all of us. We adjust our individual criteria to feel healthy in relation to others, the environment, or a particular time. Therefore, health could be defined as a balanced state in which our daily rhythms continue naturally, without the help of drugs or supplements.

The human body is a sophisticated machine with an average lifespan of 75 years. This time can often be extended another 10–15 years with good care and certain "insurance policies." But these are not the insurance policies offered by government or private health care. Rather, these policies reside within our body, mind, and spirit. We are the best judges of the daily function of each part of our body, fine-tuning each part for the best outcome. Each unit of our body's cells is a complete set of tools to function and survive. These units thrive in a community — the body — where higher-order structure and division of labor allow for specialized functions as well as the functioning of the system as a whole. Cells specialize in specific functions through a process called differentiation. This process allows different cells with a similar basic structure to acquire unique capabilities; for example, heart muscle cells can beat, skeletal muscle cells can contract and stretch, and pancreatic cells can produce insulin. These specialized functions network with each other, and the right amount of networking provides balance to the body, which can be thought of as health or a good quality of life.

To study how cells work, scientists can grow or "culture" human cells in the laboratory. Like cells in the body, cultured cells can have highly differentiated functions. The beating of heart muscle cells, the insulin secretion of pancreatic cells, the neurite outgrowth of brain cells, the formation of myotubes from muscle cells, and the migration of cancer cells have all been well documented in cultured cells. Remarkably, cultured cells can also mimic the aging process. Most normal cells divide only a limited number of times before entering a permanent state of growth arrest, even when the cells have sufficient nutrients, growth factors, and space to grow. This feature of limited replicative capacity is called senescence and is an excellent model for understanding many aspects of aging.

Old or senescent cells change their shape and function, altering their ability to cope with stress. Analyses of genetic material and proteins show that aging in individual cells, as in whole organisms, is characterized by complex structural and functional changes in molecules and their interactions. These same changes occur in cultured cells — when stressed, they enter early senescence. This provides evidence that stress is a major contributor to aging. Research on stress provides a good way to develop interventions for aging that add "life to years" and not just "years to life" to the human lifespan.

Cancer cells are an important tool for studying cellular processes and changes. Unlike cultured normal cells, which divide only a certain number of times, cancer cells divide continuously in culture and can be frozen and grown indefinitely. This allows researchers to use cultured cancer cells to study their biology and develop drugs to treat cancer. Remarkably, just like older people, old cells are more likely to become cancerous. In addition, old cells accumulate and secrete molecules that increase the likelihood that neighboring young cells will also become cancerous.

Our research laboratory studies the molecular biology of stress and aging using cultured cells. Through many years of research, our laboratory has identified two proteins that are important in how cells respond to stress: mortalin and collaborator of ARF (abbreviated CARF). Mortalin has multiple functions and is essential for cell survival. Cancer cells express high levels of mortalin, which allows the cells to grow continuously by inhibiting the signals that normally stop cell growth and cause cell death. Because mortalin supports the proliferation and inhibits the death of cancer cells, it has been targeted as an anti-cancer treatment. In contrast to cancer cells, aging cells have decreased levels of mortalin, which causes oxidative and molecular damage to accumulate in these cells. Oxidative damage is caused by "free radical" molecules that can cause cellular injury but are neutralized by antioxidants. Experimental and clinical models of Parkinson's and Alzheimer's diseases have shown that these diseases are associated with decreased mortalin levels. Cells in these disease models are unable to cope with oxidative damage or clear waste molecules from the cell. Thus, maintaining proper levels of mortalin is important to prevent age-related brain diseases and to combat stress. It is therefore a current challenge in our research to find strategies to maintain mortalin levels in old age as a new treatment for these diseases and to improve quality of life.

The second protein identified in our laboratory, CARF, regulates cell division by monitoring its stress levels and genetic damage. Stressed and senescent cells have high levels of CARF, which contributes to their growth arrest. Interestingly, cancer cells also have high levels of CARF, which instead helps the cancer cells divide. Stress can also increase CARF levels, causing cells to senesce prematurely or become cancerous. Amazingly, the same protein can switch its role from causing cell death or senescence to causing cancer. Thus, balance is key; while the right amount of CARF is essential for cells to divide and function, its deficiency causes them to die.

As we continued to unravel the biology of mortalin and CARF, dissecting their roles in normal and disease states and developing tools to control their expression to maintain their functions for healthy body states and disease interventions, we were inspired by the traditional knowledge of the therapeutic potential of herbs for health and balance. While a variety of botanicals have been developed into drugs to treat specific diseases, including cancer, herbal extracts have traditionally been used to promote a healthy lifespan and enhance the quality of life in normal and disease scenarios. In contrast to synthetic chemicals, herbs offer a simple and economical resource with enormous power to promote quality of life.

Ayurveda (*ayu* = life and *veda* = knowledge), literally translated as "knowledge of life," is a world-renowned traditional system of medicine from India. It originated around the 15th century BCE as the Atharvaveda system of home remedies and traveled through the next centuries by faith and word of mouth. With a history of more than 5,000 years of use, Ayurveda categorizes the human body into three types (called dosa): Vata, Pitta, and Kapha, which are attributed to a well-coordinated balance between the energies of mind, body, and spirit. Vata-type individuals have qualities of space and air, endowed with physical and mental qualities such as quick thinking and fast movement. A Pitta-type individual has characteristics of fire and water and is dominated by clarity, radiance, and aggression in thought and action. Kapha-type individuals have structural and physical aspects that tend to be cool, slow, soft, and stable.

An imbalance between the elemental energies of mind, body, and spirit in each type results in disease. Ayurvedic medicine uses herbs to cure or prevent such ailments by increasing energy and well-being, reducing stress, and balancing the mind, body, and spirit. Ayurvedic elements are often integrated into complementary and alternative medicine to treat a wide range of chronic diseases. These elements are trusted not only for their minimal side effects but also for their safety compared to the toxicity of conventional synthetic drugs, which have additional shortcomings such as high cost, single targets, and drug resistance. Herbal extracts, on the contrary, are inexpensive and widely available and have multi-target effects and low levels of drug resistance. In fact, many conventional drugs approved by the U.S. Food and Drug Administration (FDA) are derived from plants, such as morphine, atropine, eugenol, reserpine, taxol, and cisplatin. Among the thousands of medicinal plants described in Ayurveda, many are considered Jivaniya (health-promoting), Vayasthapana (anti-aging), and Brmhaniya (strengthening).

Ashwagandha (*Withania somnifera*), a highly prized plant crowned as the Queen of Ayurveda, grows in subtropical parts of the Indian subcontinent. Heavily used in health supplements for various activities, Ashwagandha has been trusted to improve the quality of life under normal and stressful conditions. Laboratories have studied the bioactivities of Ashwagandha, encouraging its use for health and disease management. Over the past decade, our laboratory has discovered and demonstrated anti-cancer activities in the leaves of Ashwagandha. We have defined the bioactivities in Ashwagandha leaf powder and demonstrated their dose-dependent effects and mechanisms. Remarkably, extracts of the plant are more potent than individual purified compounds and offer a multi-target therapy for cancer and age-related diseases, including Parkinson's and Alzheimer's. With the goal of improving quality of life, we sought to understand how Ashwagandha bioactivity works and to develop technologies to produce extracts with maximum and multi-target activity. We integrated and leveraged the strengths of traditional knowledge of herbal potentials, modern technologies including bioinformatics and molecular signaling, and young talent from India and Japan.

In this book, we attempt to portray the bioactivities as well as the pharmacological and therapeutic value of Ashwagandha, which has been supported by research laboratories worldwide. We wish to translate laboratory knowledge into a general understanding with the hope of bringing the benefits of Ashwagandha to human health and quality of life in normal and disease scenarios, especially in the aging population.

About the Authors

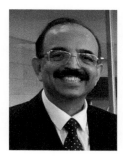

Dr. Sunil Kaul was born and raised in Kalimpong (Darjeeling), India. He received his MPhil and PhD degrees from the University of Delhi, India. After initial post-doctoral training, he was appointed as a researcher at the National Institute of Advanced Industrial Science & Technology (AIST) in Japan, where he has been working for the past 34 years. His main research interest is to understand the molecular mechanism of stress, aging, and cancer. He has merged traditional knowledge with modern technologies, like gene silencing and imaging, to understand the mechanism of action of the Ayurvedic herb, Ashwagandha, in particular. With more than 245 research publications in international peer-reviewed journals and several invited lectures internationally, he has been on the editorial board of several scientific journals. He is the chairman of the Indian Scientists Association in Japan (ISAJ), a registered non-profit organization (NPO) in Japan. He is the president of KAUL-Tech Co. Ltd., Japan (an AIST-based venture) and research advisor of ReHeva BioSciences, USA. He has served as a professor at the University of Tsukuba (Japan) and Hanyang University (Korea). He has been honored as a fellow of the Geriatrics Society of India (FGSI), an overseas fellow of the Biotech Research Society of India (FBRSI), a fellow of the Indian Academy of Neuroscience (FIAN), and a foreign fellow of the National Academy of Sciences, India (FNASI).

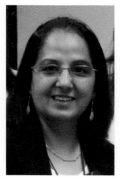

Dr. Renu Wadhwa received her first PhD from Guru Nanak Dev University, India, and her second PhD from the University of Tsukuba, Japan. She did her post-doctoral training at the University of Newcastle Upon Tyne, England, and RIKEN, Japan. She has been working in Japan for the past 33 years and is leading a research team working on the mechanisms of cell proliferation control at the Cellular and Molecular Biotechnology Research Institute (CMB), AIST, Japan. Her main research interest is to understand the molecular mechanism of aging and cancer using normal and cancer cells as a model system. She first cloned a novel member of the hsp70 family protein in 1993 and named it "mortalin." Since then, she has made several original discoveries describing the functional properties of this protein and its role in cancer and age-related diseases. She has more than 270 publications in international peer-reviewed journals with many invited/plenary talks at international conferences. She has been a member of AACR (1997–2000) and president of the 86th Annual Meeting of the Japanese Tissue Culture Association at AIST Tsukuba and was a leader of the DBT-AIST International Laboratory for Advanced Biomedicine (DAILAB) at AIST, Japan (2013–2021). She has served on the editorial boards of several scientific journals, including the *Journal of Gerontology: Biological Sciences* and *Mechanism of Aging and Development*. In honorary academic positions, she has served as an associate professor at the University of Tokyo, a professor at Yonsei University College of Medicine, Seoul, and a professor at Hanyang University, Seoul. She is presently a professor at the School of Integrative and Global Majors (SIGMA), University of Tsukuba, Japan. She is a fellow of the Geriatric Society of India, the Indian Academy of Neurosciences, the Biotech Research Society, India, and fellow of National Academy of Sciences, India.

1 What Is Ashwagandha? What Does It Have?

Ashwagandha (*Withania somnifera*) – also called Indian ginseng, Wonder Shrub, Winter Cherry, and Queen of Ayurveda – is the most valued medicinal plant in Ayurveda. The name *Ashwagandha* comes from the Sanskrit language and is a combination of two words: *Ashwa* means horse and *gandha* means smell. It refers to the strong "horse-like" odor of Ashwagandha roots and the "horse-like" power it imparts to the body's physical and mental functions. The species name *somnifera* means sleep-inducing and relaxing, which is widely recognized in Ayurveda. The genus *Withania* contains more than 23 species that are widely distributed in tropical and subtropical areas such as the arid regions of Africa, South Asia, and Central Asia, especially India, Bangladesh, Pakistan, Afghanistan, Sri Lanka, Egypt, Morocco, and South Africa.

The plant is an evergreen, woody, branched shrub that grows 30–90 cm tall, with branched stems bearing rich green leaves. The leaves are simple and oval-shaped, arranged in an alternating pattern on the stems of the plant. The space between the leaf branch and the stem contains a cluster of 5–25 pale green flowers. The flowers are small (4–6 mm in diameter) and are attached to small stems. The petals are totally or partially fused into a tube. The fruit (berry) is green when unripe and turns orange-red when ripe, enclosing numerous small seeds. The roots are light brown, extensively branched, cylindrical, and very strong (Figure 1.1).

Commonly known as Rasayana in Ayurveda, where its use can be traced back to at least 6000 BC, Ashwagandha is believed to promote a youthful and balanced state of mind and body, with a wide range of pharmaceutical and nutraceutical properties. With an annual consumption of ~12,000 tons, it has been listed as one of the 32 most sought-after medicinal plants in the world by the National Medicinal Plant Board of India. In India, Ashwagandha is widely cultivated in the states of Punjab, Madhya Pradesh, Uttar Pradesh, and Gujarat. Almost all parts of Ashwagandha are used for health benefits. The growth cycle from seed to fruit is shown in Figure 1.2.

The pharmacological properties of any plant depend on its bioactive constituents, called phytochemicals. Since Ashwagandha has been relied upon for a wide range of health-promoting activities in Ayurveda, laboratories have studied and reported various compounds, called metabolites, produced in the leaves and roots of the plant. At least 48 primary and secondary metabolites from roots and 62 from leaves have been reported. These include compounds with both health-promoting and pharmacological activities, such as alkaloids, flavonoids, steroidal lactones (withanolides), saponins, tannins, terpenoids, tropins, sitoindosides, and sterols. The majority of these compounds are 1-oxo steroids and/or are oxidized at C-26 and C-22 or C-26 and C-23 to form a β- or α-lactone. Some of these are 14 α-hydroxy steroids, 4-OH

DOI: 10.1201/9781032705743-1

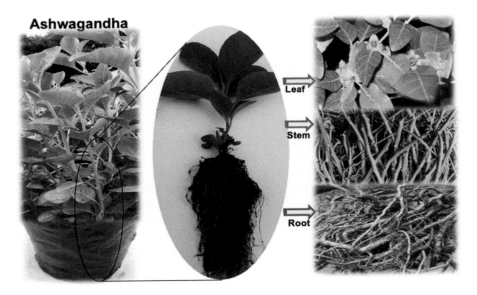

FIGURE 1.1 Images of Ashwagandha plants (left), young twigs (center), and mature leaves with berries (right-top), stem (right center), and root (right bottom).

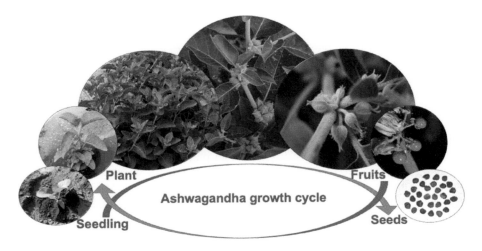

FIGURE 1.2 The growth cycle of Ashwagandha from seedling to fruit to seed.

and 5, 6-epoxy withanolides (withaferin A-like steroids) and 5-OH and 6, 7-epoxy withanolides (withanolides A and D-like steroids), 12-deoxy withastramonolide, and 14, 15β-epoxy withanolide I and 17β-hydroxy withanolide K (Figure 1.3).

Among the various phytochemicals found in Ashwagandha, withanolides are the most important pharmaceutical constituents. These compounds have diverse

Ashwagandha phytochemicals

- 1-oxo-22R-witha-2, 14-24-
- 2, 24-dienolide (Steroidal lactone)
- 3α-methoxy-2, 3-dihydro-
- 4β, 17α-dihydroxy-1-1oxo-
- 4β-dihydroxy-5β, 6β-epoxy-
- 5β, 6β-epoxy-22R-witha-
- 7-hydroxywithanolide
- 27-deoxywithaferin A (Steroidal lactone)
- Ashwagandhanolide
- Sitoindosides VII (Acylsteryl-glucoside)
- Sitoindosides VIII (Acylsteryl-glucoside)
- Sitoindosides IX (Glycowithanolide)
- Sitoindosides X (Glycowithanolide)
- Trienolide (steroidal lactone)
- Withaferin (Steroidal lactone)
- Withaferin A (Steroidal lactone)
- Withanine (Alkaloid)
- Withananine (Alkaloid)
- Withanolide A
- Withanolide B
- Withanolide D (Steroidal lactone)
- Withanolide E (Steroidal lactone)
- Withanolide - WS 2 (Aliphatic ester)
- Withanolide - WS 1 (Aliphatic ketone)
- Withanone (Steroidal lactone)

FIGURE 1.3   List of major phytochemicals found in Ashwagandha.

biological activities and give Ashwagandha an earthy odor. They are structurally similar to the active compounds found in Asian ginseng (*Panax ginseng*), which is why Ashwagandha is also known as Indian ginseng. Withaferin A was the first withanolide reported in 1965, and, since then, over the past 50 years, 1,000 withanolides have been discovered from the scientific plant families of Solanaceae, Leguminosae, Labiatae, Myrtaceae, and Taccaceae. Withanone, withanolide A, withanolide E, and withanolide D are important bioactive compounds with disease-preventive and therapeutic value.

Withanolides are synthesized in the roots and leaves of plants, with concentrations varying from 0.001% to 2.0% in different parts of the plant. Furthermore, leaves and roots have different profiles of secondary metabolites. Withaferin A and withanone are mainly found in leaves, while roots are the major site of withanolide A. Withaferin A increases in leaves and roots as young (6 weeks old) to mature (12–18 weeks old) plants grow, followed by a decrease in withanolides as plants continue to mature. Roots also contain alkaloids (withanaminine, pseudowithamine, somniferinine, withanine, somniferine, somnine, withananine, pseudowithanine, tropine, 3-a-gloyloxytropane, choline, cuscohygrine, isopelletierine, and anaferine andanahydrine), acylsteryl glucosides (sitoindosides VII and VIII), and glycowithanolides (sitoindosides IX and X). The leaves contain steroidal lactones (withaferin, withaferin A, withanolide D, withanolide E, withanone, 27-deoxywithaferin A, trienolide, and 2,24-dienolide), withanolide B, withanolide Z, and 7-hydroxywithanolide. Ashwagandhanolide, a bioactive dimeric thiowithanolide compound, has also been isolated from Ashwagandha.

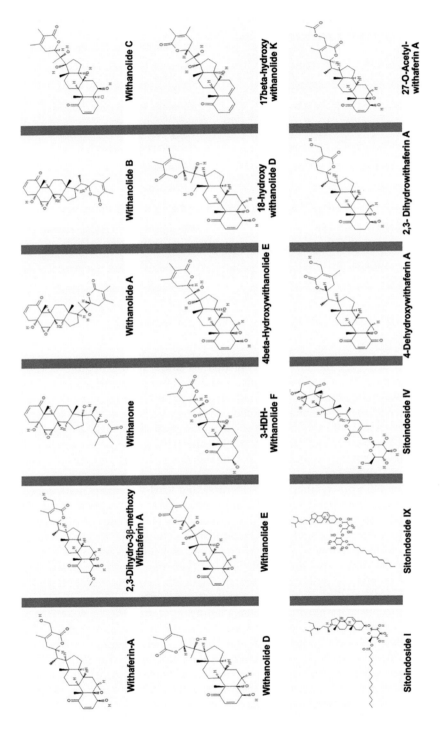

FIGURE 1.4   Structure of the major phytochemicals found in Ashwagandha.

2 What Is Ashwagandha Known for?

Longevity and Rejuvenation; Sharp Memory, Intellect, and Cognitive Power; Freedom from Disease; Strength of a Horse

Ashwagandha, long trusted and proudly known as the Queen of Ayurveda, is the most widely used herb for improving quality of life. Only recently have laboratories tested the plant's bioactivities in cell and animal experiments, further encouraging the use of Ashwagandha to manage health and disease. These laboratory studies have supported several established functions of Ashwagandha. An overview of these activities is shown in Figure 2.1 and summarized below. For additional details, the reader is encouraged to consult the detailed scientific reports.

- Ayurveda describes the use of Ashwagandha for rejuvenation. Laboratory studies using either cultured cells or animal models support that extracts from the whole plant or various parts (roots, stems, leaves, and bark) possess health-promoting, disease-preventing, and therapeutic activities. Reported activities include anti-stress, anti-inflammatory, anti-microbial, anti-arthritic, anti-diabetic, anti-leishmanial, anti-ischemic, hypoxia-modulating, anti-cancer, cardioprotective, neuroprotective, and immuno-modulatory activities associated with rejuvenation.
- As indicated by its species name, *somnifera*, Ashwagandha contains high levels of withanolides and has a sleep-inducing effect.
- Often referred to as the herb of Aphrodite (after the Greek goddess of beauty and sexual attractiveness), Ashwagandha is believed to increase sexual desire. This reputation is because it works in a variety of ways to enrich the physical and mental well-being of the body, which is likely related to pleasurable sexual experiences. The inability to enjoy sexual pleasure is associated with fatigue and nervous exhaustion; Ashwagandha promotes calmness and restfulness, which may account for its aphrodisiac activity.

DOI: 10.1201/9781032705743-2

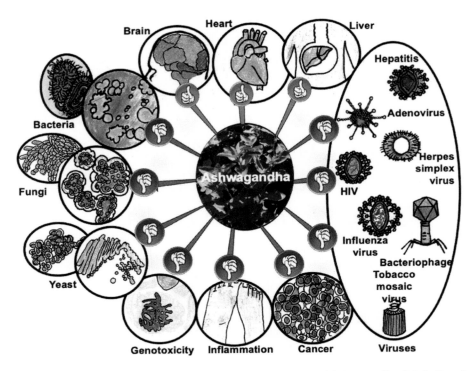

FIGURE 2.1 Pictorial representation of the known activities of Ashwagandha. It is believed to be good for brain, heart, and liver function (top) and blocks the growth of microorganisms (bacteria, fungi, and yeast) (left). It protects against genetic damage, inflammation, cancer, and a variety of viruses (bottom and right).

- Ashwagandha acts on the hypothalamic–pituitary–adrenal hormonal and signaling axis, as well as the neuroendocrine system, which controls how our body responds to stress. Thus, Ashwagandha induces a state of harmony between various physiological functions.
- Ashwagandha's adaptogenic properties – its ability to promote balance in the body and help manage stress – are the result of the combined beneficial functions of several potent withanolides, alkaloids, and other compounds. Preclinical research and clinical studies support the therapeutic use of this plant to improve cardiovascular function, liver function, and cognitive and memory-related disorders.

Most of the initial research has explored the potential benefits of root extracts of Ashwagandha or its active ingredients, and traditional home medicine has also focused on Ashwagandha roots. But why? We investigated by measuring the major bioactive components of withanolides in Ashwagandha roots and leaves. To our surprise, we measured 20 times higher levels of major withanolides in leaves compared to roots. So why were the roots traditionally used in home medicine? Was the low level in roots considered sufficient? Or were roots thought to be purer because they grow underground?

Harvesting roots requires destroying the plant to obtain low levels of active ingredients. Instead, one could easily pick the leaves to get higher concentrations of the same compounds and also maintain the plants for several harvests. In addition, the roots are extremely strong, deeply rooted, and difficult to harvest and clean. Concerns such as contamination with soil bacteria make it difficult to establish roots as a quality-controlled food.

To understand these factors, we asked several Ayurvedic practitioners why they focus on Ashwagandha roots. They indicated that, in addition to the fact that the root has historically been considered pure, the main reason is that the roots are easier to dry than the leaves. Roots are solid and heavy, so it is convenient to leave them outdoors to dry in the sun. They are not blown away, and wild animals will not eat the roots because of their strong smell, so processing is easy. Leaves, on the contrary, contain large amounts of water, attract mold during the drying process, and must be protected from wind and wild animals. While drying in electric machines such as dehydrators is an obvious solution today, this was not an option in the past. Interestingly, when we asked practitioners if they knew about the active ingredients and their content in different parts of the plant, the answers were vague. No one had actually researched the active compounds of Ashwagandha and their mechanisms of action. Because word of mouth was so strong, no one was looking for scientific evidence.

Trends have gradually changed over time, and it is only in the past few decades that herbs and herbal extracts have been brought into the laboratory to validate their effects and understand how they work. However, this testing has been successful – about 40% of FDA-approved drugs for cancer treatment are derived from herbs. These include cisplatin, paclitaxel, vincristine, vinblastine, and thymoquinone. However, all of these drugs have adverse side effects, unlike the parent plants from which they are derived. This suggests that the plants must contain other components that protect the cells from toxicity.

Because different parts of the Ashwagandha plant have different active ingredients, it is often the case that individual parts of the plant are prescribed for specific purposes.

The roots contain withanolide A and withanolide D as major metabolites. They have a peculiar horsey smell and are traditionally recommended for the treatment of ulcers, pimples, pain, swelling, worms, hemorrhoids, constipation, rheumatism, arthritis, leucoderma, insomnia, nervous breakdowns, goiter, and cognitive and psychomotor abnormalities. Roots strengthen and calm the nervous system. Taken over time, they can help build up emaciated tissues, reduce negative reactions to stress, and increase energy levels. The leaves contain withaferin A and withanone as major metabolites. They have a bitter taste and smell similar to green tea. Leaves are recommended as a general tonic and rejuvenator for good physical and mental health, as a stress reliever, and for anti-aging, antioxidant, anti-inflammatory, anti-cancer, and anti-diabetic activities. They also treat fever, worms, pain, inflammation, and high blood pressure. The flowers are used for their aphrodisiac and diuretic properties. The seeds are anthelmintic, which means they are used to treat worms. They are mixed with rock salt and used to remove white spots from the cornea. Seeds are also used to treat hysteria, memory loss, and anxiety and to increase sperm count.

We were curious about how one herb could have so many beneficial effects. So, with this basic knowledge of the plant and its ancient uses, our lab explored Ashwagandha's power against stress, aging, and cancer. We were clear about the following:

- We wanted to avoid a biased approach, such as testing an already-reported effect in another experimental model. Instead, we wanted to discover the full potential of Ashwagandha.
- We wanted in-depth research to solve the centuries-old mystery of Ashwagandha's effects.
- We wanted to avoid conclusions from our research that were not supported by mechanisms of action.
- We wanted to learn about Ashwagandha by testing all of the plant's constituents, rather than picking and choosing specific ones.

We wondered if one condition could cause several others and if Ashwagandha could treat this underlying condition. After much discussion, we thought that Ashwagandha's effects might be stress-related, so we began our journey with stress models. Like us, cells experience stress and respond by altering the proteins they produce – increasing the expression of stress proteins to cope with the changes, while turning down the expression of proteins used for normal cell function to conserve energy. We began with experiments on cultured cells to test whether Ashwagandha has preventive or therapeutic power in times of stress.

Because Ashwagandha's active compounds are variable throughout the plant, we debated how to approach our experiments – do we take a reductionist approach to test individual compounds, or do we take a holistic approach to gain the benefits of crude herbal extracts rather than purified individual compounds? And which part of the plant to choose – the tough roots with low concentrations of active compounds or the tender leaves with higher concentrations?

We decided to use the leaves because we could collect an abundant supply without sacrificing the whole plant. Because we wanted to understand the holistic effects of Ashwagandha, we made a variety of extracts using different solvents, including organic solvents, alcohol, and water. We used these extracts to test Ashwagandha's activity in our cell models to answer questions about stress intervention, aging, cancer, and cell differentiation, comparing our data to what is known in traditional home medicine.

3 What Are the Major Active Ingredients of Ashwagandha, and What Do They Do?
Scientific Validity

Herbs have attracted much attention in the global healthcare sector, and there has been an increasing investment in traditional herbal medicine research in the past two decades. As described in the last chapter, our first series of homework toward the long-term goals to obtain scientific validation of the well-trusted benefits of Ashwagandha, led us to research its leaves. At times, we also used roots and compared their activities with that of leaves. Cell culture models, very fascinating and fast, had one limitation unlike the animal models and human beings – we cannot make them eat the herbal powders. Like infants, they can be fed only on a liquid diet and that too water-based. So the leaf and root extracts made in organic solvent or alcohol were to be diluted to the extent that cells do not sense the organic solvents at all. A particular hurdle we faced when testing Ashwagandha extracts was variation in their contents. In fact, we struggled to standardize methods to produce a uniform Ashwagandha leaf extract. This alerted us that the plant itself had variability in its components, which could be due to plant variety, the soil it grows in, varying environmental conditions (such as light, moisture, and minerals), stage of growth, microbial environment, or other factors. Because the bioactive compounds (withanolides) are produced in the plant for its defense, we could easily relate variability to environmental conditions. This also alerted us that the various commercially available Ashwagandha products would differ in their contents and likely have large batch-to-batch variations.

We examined ~30 Ashwagandha products sold in the market with a variety of fancy labels. None of these defined what they contained beyond the "Ashwagandha" name. There was hardly any description of which part of the plant was used or what active ingredients it contained. This stoked our motivation to establish scientifically validated Ashwagandha products with defined chemical signatures and bioactivities. We aimed to produce extracts for holistic activity, with minimal side effects and maximal benefits – which was not an easy task to achieve with comprehensive scientific validation.

We began with a reductionist approach. We needed to define the active ingredients and their activities both individually and in combination. Then, we needed to generate natural and artificial combinations and test them in the laboratory. Modern medical

DOI: 10.1201/9781032705743-3

drugs developed with chemicals have dramatically improved human health and therapeutics. These medical drugs have become part of a comfortable life in developed countries. At the same time, many synthetic drugs have adverse effects, including toxicity to the liver and/or heart. We often even hear on the news when drugs are withdrawn from the market. In clinical trials, 40%–50% of drugs in development are terminated because they are not effective or are very toxic. And, in addition to the extremely high cost of drug development, drug availability and affordability are hurdles once new drugs enter the market. At the same time, many ailments still have limited treatment options, with either no drugs or no accessibility to existing drugs. We felt that our reductionist approach to dissecting and understanding the chemistry and biology of active natural ingredients would best align with the potential usage of these compounds.

Here we describe some basic research on the molecular mechanisms of Ashwagandha activities from laboratories worldwide. Interested readers are advised to refer to the specific research papers and our scientific book (Kaul and Wadhwa, 2017) for further information. Specific bioactivities of some of the many withanolides in Ashwagandha have been determined from experiments using either cultured cells or rodent models. Here we list some of the main activities of withaferin A, withanone, withanolide A, withanolide D, and withanolide E that have been validated in the laboratory.

3.1   WITHAFERIN A

- Inhibits the growth of various cancer cells including human breast carcinoma (both estrogen-responsive and irresponsive), myeloma, endothelial carcinoma, osteosarcoma, pancreatic carcinoma, glioblastoma, neuroblastoma, lymphoblastic leukemia, and oral squamous cell carcinoma.
- Reduces the growth of tumors significantly in mouse models.
- Inhibits the ability of cancer cells to spread from a tumor to other parts of the body, called metastasis, and develop new blood vessels, called angiogenesis, in mouse models.
- Reduces the expression of intercellular adhesion molecule-1 (ICAM1) and vascular cell adhesion molecule-1 (VCAM-1), proteins important for interactions between cells, tumor progression, and metastasis.
- Suppresses tumor growth in mouse models of pancreatic cancer.
- Anti-inflammatory effects in inflammatory disorders such as rheumatoid arthritis and airway inflammation in various disease models.
- Reduces inflammation in rabbit cartilage cells by upregulating the expression of the enzyme cyclooxygenase-2 (COX-2).
- Inhibits the activity of enzymes that break down proteins and cause tumor regression in mouse models of malignant lung mesothelioma.
- Inhibits angiogenesis by blocking the activity of a protein called vascular endothelial growth factor and thereby reduces tumor mass and lung metastasis in mouse models of cancer.
- Activates the p53 tumor suppressor protein, stopping the growth of tumor cells.

- Inactivates processes that promote malignant properties of cancer cells, including rapid proliferation, migration, and invasion, by reducing the expression of several proteins including uPA (extracellular matrix-degrading protease), PLAT (plasminogen activator), ADAM8 (a disintegrin and metalloprotease-8), integrins, laminins, TNFSF12 (tumor necrosis factor superfamily member 12), interleukin 6 (IL-6), ANGPTL2 (angiopoietin-like protein 2), CSF1R (colony-stimulating factor 1 receptor), and mortalin.
- Suppresses proteins that determine cancer cell metastasis and angiogenesis including, vimentin, MMP-9 (matrix metalloproteinases-9), and Akt or protein kinase B signaling causing inhibition of epithelial-to-mesothelial transition in breast and ovarian cancer cells.

3.2 WITHANOLIDE A

- Has strong pharmacological action, especially related to the nervous system.
- Targets and blocks β-amyloid deposition in the brain, which is thought to be responsible for Alzheimer's disease, in rat models. It does this by targeting multiple proteins like BACE1, an aspartic-acid protease involved in the formation of myelin sheaths, ADAM10 (a disintegrin and metalloprotease-10), IDE (insulin-degrading enzyme) and NEP (neprilysin).
- Has neuroprotective ability with its potential to inhibit the enzyme cholinesterase, which breaks down chemical signaling molecules in the brain called neurotransmitters.
- Reduces epileptic seizures.
- Improves memory impairment.
- Recovers degeneration of neurons and loss of the junctions between neurons, which are important for how neurons communicate with one another.
- Combats various nervous system pathologies, especially related to Alzheimer's disease.
- Recover immune system function by normalizing T cells, which play a central role in the immune response.

3.3 WITHANOLIDE D

- Has anti-fungal, anti-bacterial, and anti-oxidant activities.
- Prevents damage to the liver.
- Has adaptogenic activity, meaning that it is a plant compound that helps the body handle stress.
- Has anti-inflammatory and anti-stress activities.
- Causes growth arrest and cell death in various cultured human cancer cells including pancreatic ductal adenocarcinoma cells, estrogen-responsive and irresponsive breast carcinoma, myeloma, lymphoma, epidermoid carcinoma, and nasopharynx carcinoma.
- Inhibits the growth of highly malignant human sarcoma in mouse models.

3.4   WITHANOLIDE E

- Inhibits the proliferation of human pancreatic and breast cancer cells in both a culture dish and mice models.
- Inhibits the activity of the overreactive immune system.
- Suppresses the proliferation of T and B lymphocytes, which are the main components of the immune response to specific pathogens.

3.5   WITHANONE

- Prevents the growth of various cultured human cancer cells.
- Inhibits tumor growth and metastasis in immunosuppressed mouse models.
- Has anti-stress and anti-aging activities in normal cells.
- Induces cultured brain-derived cells to differentiate into glial and neural cells.
- Protects against memory loss and stress in cell cultures and mouse models.

3.6   COMBINATIONS PROVE TO BE POWERFUL

Several studies have shown that the effect of two combined compounds of Ashwagandha is more beneficial than each compound.

- Withaferin A, combined with either withanone or withanolide A, causes better differentiation of brain-derived cells in culture compared to each of the compounds alone.
- Withaferin A, combined with sorafenib, a clinically approved drug to treat renal cell carcinoma, is better at killing specific cancer cells than either compound alone. This combination had potent anti-cancer activity at low doses of sorafenib, which is promising for its potential use in cancer treatment.
- Withaferin A, combined with cisplatin, a chemotherapy drug, reduces tumor growth by up to 70%–80% and completely inhibits cancer metastasis in immunosuppressed mice compared to untreated mice and mice treated only with cisplatin.
- Since withaferin A helps kill human lymphoma cells when treated with ionizing radiation, it has been proposed as a sensitizer to enhance the effect of radiation therapy.
- A natural derivative of withaferin A that is structurally similar (3-dihydro-3β-methoxy withaferin A) is found in alcohol extracts of Ashwagandha leaves. In contrast to withaferin A, its derivative does not have anti-cancer and anti-metastasis activities. However, the derivative protects normal cells against a variety of stresses (oxidative, UV radiation, and chemical), suggesting that a mixture of withaferin A and its derivative might kill cancer cells but be safe for normal cells. Such a combination could offer safer and milder chemotherapy.

4 What Are the Bioactivities of Ashwagandha?
Extracts, Experiments, and Evidence

We hypothesized that the beneficial health effects of Ashwagandha might be due to its anti-stress activity and set out to investigate this experimentally. For simplicity, stress can be divided into two main categories: (i) oxidative stress, which primarily affects protein structure and function, and (ii) DNA damage, which affects genetic material. Before experimentally testing Ashwagandha's activities, we investigated what bioactivities were already known and whether they were related to protection against stress. The relatively extensive results are presented here as an overview, although readers should refer to the published research articles and our book (Kaul and Wadhwa, 2017) for more details.

4.1 ANTI-MUTAGENIC EFFECT

Mutagens are physical or chemical agents that alter our genetic material, DNA. These genetic changes alter the structure and function of the resulting proteins and are associated with diseases, including cancer. Agents that specifically increase the risk of cancer are called carcinogens. We encounter mutagens and carcinogens in our daily lives. Many are the result of the phenomenal growth of the chemical industry in recent decades, which has brought immense social and economic progress but also environmental contamination. In addition, lifestyle changes and the widespread use of synthetic chemicals and plastics have reduced environmental quality, contributing to negative health effects. Exposure to environmental pollutants damages human DNA and increases the risk of health problems such as high blood pressure, reduced kidney function, cognitive disorders, cancer, and even death. Protecting people from overexposure to environmental mutagens and carcinogens is a major challenge today.

To determine whether a substance is a mutagen, it is important to know how much of a health risk it poses at a given concentration. Because direct testing in humans is not feasible for logistical, ethical, and practical reasons, tests using experimental models of bacteria, insects, plants, human cell cultures, and animals are employed to study environmental contaminants. Many research laboratories use a simple test

DOI: 10.1201/9781032705743-4

called the onion root chromosome aberration assay to test how substances affect genetic material. The World Health Organization recommends the assay as a reliable and economical way to test for environmental mutagens. The assay is also used to test the genetic effects of plant extracts rich in bioactive compounds called phytochemicals.

For example, researchers tested whether Ashwagandha leaf extract could protect against genetic defects caused by a mutagen called N-methyl-N'-nitro-N-nitrosoguanidine (MNNG). MNNG causes several genetic defects, including abnormal aggregation of chromosomes during cell division. These are technically defined as c-mitosis, stickiness, delayed anaphases, laggards, wandering chromosomes, chromatid bridges, and chromosome breaks. In a standard assay, germinating onion root tips are exposed to MNNG to induce the cytogenetic abnormalities described above. They are then treated with Ashwagandha to determine the level of protection and recovery. Treatment with Ashwagandha leaf extract was found to provide ~90% protection against MNNG-induced cytogenetic defects. This effect occurs regardless of whether the extract is applied concurrently, before, or after treatment with MNNG.

Experiments in rats exposed to lead showed that treatment with Ashwagandha leaf extract reduced genetic defects (micronucleated polychromatic erythrocytes) induced by lead exposure. These experiments suggest that Ashwagandha protects genetic material from the mutagenic effects of potent chemicals (Figure 4.1).

4.2   ANTI-MICROBIAL ACTIVITY

Microbes are tiny living organisms, often invisible to the naked eye. They include bacteria, viruses, fungi, algae, and protozoa. Microbes are found everywhere, including soil, water, and air. They are important for decomposition, climate change, and nutrient cycling. Some bacteria are essential components of our food, such as bread, cheese, and wine. Fermented foods such as kimchi, miso, natto, tempeh, pickles, sauerkraut, kombucha, kefir, and yogurt also contain microbes. Fermented foods have positive health benefits such as boosting the immune system, improving digestion, fighting bad bacteria, and reducing the risk of diseases such as cancer. The human body is also host to millions of microbes, collectively called the human microbiota or the human microbiome. These organisms are found on our skin, hair, and nails; in our nose, mouth, and ears; and inside our bodies, where they play important roles in bodily functions. For example, some microbes help with digestion, while others fight bad bacteria.

Changes in the microbiota in the upper respiratory tract, gut, and reproductive system have been linked to health problems such as allergies, infections, and even cancer. In addition, while some bacteria are necessary for normal body functions, "bad bacteria" can lead to problems such as coughing, congestion, vomiting, diabetes, obesity, cardiovascular disease, and brain disease.

Antibacterials are substances that kill bacteria and prevent them from growing. These important parts of our daily lives include soap, shampoo, and mouthwash, as well as dishwashing, laundry, and cleaning products. However, most antibiotics kill

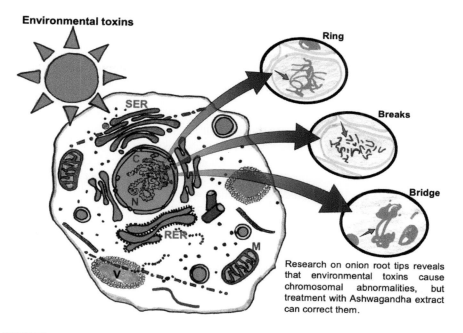

Research on onion root tips reveals that environmental toxins cause chromosomal abnormalities, but treatment with Ashwagandha extract can correct them.

FIGURE 4.1 Graphic representation of a human cell with its subcellular structures including the nucleus (N-green) containing genetic material in chromosomes (C-blue thread-like structures in the nucleus), endoplasmic reticulum (ER – blue and red), mitochondria (M-light and dark blue ladder-like structures), vacuoles (V-organs), etc. Environmental toxins cause damage to our genetic material. Stressed/damaged chromosomes show defects such as ring and bridge-like structures formed by breakage and misjoining of chromosomes. Ashwagandha extract protects against such defects.

both good and bad bacteria, which can lead to illness. It is important to maintain a balance of good bacteria in our bodies. One way to do this is to avoid antibiotics that kill all bacteria and instead use foods and herbs with specific antibiotic activity. Studies such as those listed below show that Ashwagandha compounds can kill some bad bacteria and may even tip the microbial balance toward the good.

- In traditional medicine, Ashwagandha leaves are used to treat abscesses (an infection of the hair follicle that collects pus) and carbuncles (a red, swollen, painful cluster of boils). Withaferin A (Wi-A) has antibiotic activity against some bacteria and disease-causing fungi. Studies of mice fed Ashwagandha fruit extract show that it can eliminate infection with *Salmonella* bacteria.
- Ashwagandha leaf extract also provides protection or immunity against infections caused by various viruses, protozoa, and other parasites. In studies using a mouse model of malaria (a disease caused by a protozoan transmitted by mosquitoes), treatment with Ashwagandha caused a ~50% reduction in the number of protozoa in infected mice.

- Ashwagandha root extracts have been shown to kill strains of multidrug-resistant bacteria, such as *Staphylococcus aureus*, that are resistant to conventional antibacterial drugs. Ashwagandha extracts were effective in treating bacterial and fungal infections of the skin, upper respiratory tract, gastrointestinal tract, and urinary tract.
- Ashwagandha has been shown to have anti-leishmanial activity. Leishmaniasis is caused by *Leishmania* (protozoan) parasites transmitted by the bite of infected female sandflies and has an annual incidence of 700,000–1 million new cases. The disease is associated with malnutrition, weak immune systems, and poor housing. Of the three known types of leishmaniasis, visceral (also called kala-azar) is the most severe form of the disease, with both cutaneous and mucocutaneous manifestations. Visceral leishmaniasis, one of the most important parasitic diseases, is characterized by weight loss, enlargement of the spleen and liver, irregular fevers, and anemia. Cutaneous leishmaniasis is the most common form of leishmaniasis. It causes skin lesions or ulcers on exposed parts of the body, resulting in lifelong scarring. Mucocutaneous leishmaniasis destroys the mucous membranes of the nose, mouth, and throat. In one study, extracts from ten plants commonly used in traditional home medicine in India were tested for anti-*Leishmania* activity. The extract from only two plants (Ashwagandha and garlic) showed significant activity against *Leishmania* (Figure 4.2).

Treatment of infected mice with a combination of *Asparagus racemosus* and Ashwagandha extracts not only successfully reduced parasite levels but also generated protective immune responses with the normalization of biochemical and hematological tests, suggesting their role as important anti-leishmanial agents. It causes apoptotic death of the parasite by producing reactive oxygen species (ROS) from mitochondria and disrupting mitochondrial structure and function. Wi-A has also been shown to inhibit the parasite-specific enzymes (pteridine reductase 1, PTR1) that are essential for its growth and survival.

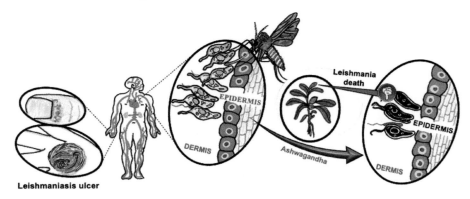

FIGURE 4.2 Schematic representation of the effect of Ashwagandha on skin ulcers caused by *Leishmania*. It is known to kill the ulcer-causing parasite and thus helps in curing the disease.

4.3 ANTI-STRESS

Any change in the environment (physical, chemical, mental, or emotional) that requires an adjustment or response from a living organism is recognized as stress. Stress is a normal part of life at all levels of organization, from cells to organisms and can be internal or external. For example, we can experience stress not only from our immediate or distant environment but also from our lifestyle, habits, or thoughts. Although stress can lead to serious conditions such as depression, anxiety, hypertension, stroke, and cancer, stress itself is not considered a disease. As a result, there are no drugs in development to treat stress. It is widely believed that we can adapt to stress or even avoid and prevent it by adjusting our lifestyles. However, mild stress is considered good because it trains and strengthens the body's defense systems. Several studies have shown that mild stress protects cells and the body from later, more intense stress. So how do we define good and bad stress? Just as we measure blood glucose to determine if we have diabetes, stress levels can probably be measured using biomarkers, including stress-specific proteins.

Some medications used to treat depression, anxiety, and panic are also available as "anti-stress" medications. These include benzodiazepines (alprazolam, clonazepam, diazepam, lorazepam, triazolam, temazepam, and chlordiazepoxide), serotonin inhibitors, sedatives (antihistamines, also used for allergic reactions), and sleep aids (glutethimide and methylprylon). These drugs suppress the activity of the central nervous system (brain and spinal cord). This has a calming effect by activating neurotransmitters such as gamma-aminobutyric acid (GABA), a natural nerve signaling molecule. However, these drugs also have side effects such as drowsiness, blurred vision, sedation, nausea, headache, diarrhea or severe constipation, drowsiness, confusion, sexual dysfunction, memory loss, and uncoordinated speech. Taking an anti-stress medication with these side effects could never be a path of choice. In fact, it can be suicidal.

Given the existing experimental evidence that mild stress can have beneficial effects, perhaps one should strive to train the body better with mild stress but avoid increasing stress to levels that require medication. The other option is to increase the buffering capacity of our bodies naturally. In traditional homeopathy, Ashwagandha has been hailed as a calming herb and rasayana (rejuvenator) that increases the body's physical and mental strength and promotes calmness and balance. Research on rodent stress models describes the anti-stress and antidepressant potential of Ashwagandha. These studies have concluded that the pharmacological potential of Ashwagandha is comparable to that of the antidepressant imipramine and the anti-anxiety drug lorazepam.

Research has shown that the anti-anxiety effect of Ashwagandha is due to its ability to mimic the activity of a neurotransmitter called GABA. Several research studies have shown that Ashwagandha extracts highly mimic GABA in mouse models. In a rat model of chronic stress induced by electric shock, rats develop adverse effects such as depression, glucose intolerance, sexual dysfunction, suppressed immune function, and gastric ulcers. Ashwagandha extract showed significant anti-stress effects in these rats. Another study reported that Ashwagandha root extract manages the body weight of adult humans under chronic stress conditions by regulating their eating behavior. The study also showed that the weight-managing role of root extract may be due to reduced levels of the stress hormone cortisol, as well as physiological and psychological stress.

In a chronic stress model, rats received a mild, unpredictable footshock once daily for 21 days. Ashwagandha extract administered 1 hour before the footshock resulted in reduced levels of behavioral depression as assessed by the swim test. Treatment of chronically stressed rats with Ashwagandha significantly reversed the effects of stress in a dose-dependent manner. In stressed adult mice, treatment with Ashwagandha extract also caused a reduction in stress-induced production of nitric oxide, a molecule that affects neuronal function. Several types of Ashwagandha extracts have been shown to reduce lipid peroxidation and increase antioxidant enzymes and catalase and superoxide dismutase (SOD) in the brain, liver, and kidney. These effects enhance the cells' defenses against stress-induced damage, suggesting that Ashwagandha may protect cells from toxic stress.

Rasayana is an Ayurvedic micronutrient supplement known to combat stress and promote healthy aging and longevity. Among its components, Ashwagandha is consistently reported as an essential adaptogenic and anti-stress herb that limits brain aging, improves memory, and promotes cognitive response and neuro-regeneration. Ashwagandha bioactives have been experimentally proven to be useful in neutralizing accumulated stress and achieving improved brain function and cognitive response even in a variety of neuropathological conditions including Alzheimer's and Parkinson's diseases and their associated abnormalities such as amnesia and dementia. Notably, Ashwagandha bioactives have not only been reported to protect against the risk of degenerative neuropathologies but also been found to reverse the effects of such pathologies at advanced stages in multiple ways. Protection against oxidative stress, activation of neuronal signaling, and reconstruction of neuronal networks by Ashwagandha bioactive compounds offer hope for targeted therapeutics. In addition, Ashwagandha bioactive compounds have anti-cancer properties, including inducing cell differentiation and death and inhibiting cell proliferation and invasive spread. Bioinformatics and computational evidence have begun to unravel the molecular action of specific bioactive compounds, opening new avenues for exploring Ashwagandha's activities.

In a typical laboratory experiment to understand and manipulate stress, living human cells are exposed to chemicals, toxic compounds, radiation, or other factors to study the underlying chemistry and biology of the cells. This is done using quantitative and qualitative biochemical and imaging techniques, including analysis of proteins, nucleic acids, intracellular structures [cell membrane, mitochondria, endoplasmic reticulum (ER), lysosomes, cytoskeleton, and vacuoles], and intercellular junctions. In a simplistic explanation, as also shown in Figure 4.3, stressed cells are damaged in two different areas: (i) genetic material, which experiences either single-strand or double-strand breaks, and (ii) cellular structures, such as mitochondria, ER, and others, which experience oxidative damage in their structure (Figure 4.3).

The anti-stress activities of natural compounds are generally defined by their ability to protect against these two broad categories of damage. Proteins that repair DNA (such as MRE11, NBS1, RAD50, and PARP-1) and provide antioxidant defense (such as CAT, SOD, and NRF2) also help protect against damage. Experimental data from

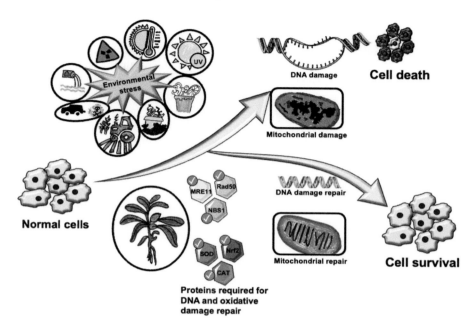

FIGURE 4.3 Schematic representation of Ashwagandha's effect against environmental stress (radiation, heat, UV, water pollution, agricultural and industrial waste, automobiles, and smoke). Most of these environmental stresses cause damage to DNA and subcellular structures including membranes and mitochondria. Ashwagandha protects against cell death caused by these stresses.

our laboratory and others show that Ashwagandha has these capabilities. Unbiased random screening for anti-stress compounds using cell culture-based approaches led to the selection of Ashwagandha constituents that have been shown to protect cells from both DNA damage and oxidative stress.

We conducted an experimental screening to identify and validate compounds with anti-stress activities that could protect against oxidative, metal, and hypoxia stresses. These stresses are known to cause many human ailments, including metabolic and cognitive disorders. We used three chemical models, namely paraquat, cadmium nitrate, and cobalt chloride, to represent these stress categories. We screened 70 compounds for their ability to protect against these stresses and selected four compounds that belonged to Ashwagandha. These compounds were Wi-A, methoxy withaferin A (mWi-A), withanone (Wi-N), and triethylene glycol (TEG). We found that stressed cells exhibited an increase in mitochondrial damage, DNA double-strand breaks, protein aggregation, and apoptosis. However, low nontoxic doses of the selected compounds provided remarkable protection against these stresses. Of note, Wi-N and TEG in combination protected against endogenous accumulation of stress validated by in vitro aging of normal human fibroblasts. The active ingredients or extracts of Ashwagandha could protect against innate stress and reduce the burden of diseases, thus enhancing the quality of life.

4.4 ANTI-INFLAMMATORY

In rat models, Ashwagandha extract showed anti-inflammatory effects in arthritic and other inflammatory conditions. It significantly reduced inflammation induced by complete Freund's adjuvant, formalin, and carrageenan (established models of inflammation that cause edema and hypersensitivity in rats). It has been shown to reduce inflammation by inhibiting cyclooxygenase, an enzyme responsible for the formation of molecules involved in inflammation. Neuroinflammation is the cause of several neurodegenerative diseases – it damages nerve cells by releasing toxic and damaging molecules and inflammatory mediators, disrupting cell membranes and mitochondria and damaging proteins. Ashwagandha extract inhibited inflammation caused by a stainless steel implant in adult zebrafish. It caused a remarkable reduction in the levels of tumor necrosis factor-alpha (TNFα) and inflammatory cytokines (Figure 4.4).

4.5 IMMUNOMODULATORY ACTIVITY

Immunomodulation, or alteration of the body's immune system by agents that affect its function, is studied in the laboratory by challenging the immune system with external stimuli such as drugs. Cyclophosphamide, azathioprine, and prednisolone

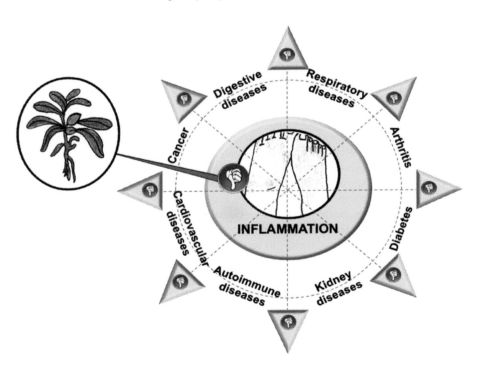

FIGURE 4.4 Ashwagandha has anti-inflammatory activity associated with a variety of diseases shown in the diagram.

are three common drugs that suppress the immune system, and hematologic and sero-logic tests monitor their effects. In mice given all three immunosuppressive drugs, treatment with Ashwagandha prevents immunosuppression. Ashwagandha-treated mice also show stimulated immune responses as monitored by a significant increase in hemolytic antibodies to foreign cells. Several independent studies have reported that Ashwagandha supplementation increases white blood cell production, inhibits delayed-type hypersensitivity reactions in mice, and stimulates the production of cytotoxic T lymphocytes. Ashwagandha extracts and the bioactive withanolide A have been shown to have immunopotentiating and myeloprotective effects by increasing levels of interferon (IFN)-γ, interleukin (IL)-2, and granulocyte–macrophage colony-stimulating factor in normal and cyclophosphamide-treated mice.

4.6 BRAIN HEALTH

Because the brain consumes a large amount of energy, it generates many ROS that contribute to brain dysfunction, such as the memory impairments that are most com-mon with aging. Ashwagandha extracts show high potential to protect the brain from oxidative stress and age-related conditions such as fatigue, stroke, dyskinesia ("trem-ors"), Parkinson's disease, Alzheimer's disease, Huntington's disease (HD), epilepsy, catalepsy, insomnia, and memory loss. In Ayurveda, Ashwagandha is considered a brain tonic and a memory and cognitive-enhancing herb. Ashwagandha is believed to provide physiological and behavioral rejuvenation.

Several research laboratories around the world have demonstrated that Ashwagandha extracts and purified components can protect cells from neurotoxic agents (such as cyclosphamide and its derivatives, kainic acid, streptozotocin, 6-hydroxydopamine, methoxyacetic acid (MAA), lead, maneb paraquat, and sco-polamine). Such activity has been attributed to bioactive compounds such as Wi-N, withanolide A, and glycowithanolides. A representative list of activities supported by laboratory data is as follows:

- Withanolide A caused significant nerve cell renewal (both axons and dendrites), restored presynapses and postsynapses, and reversed memory loss caused by β-amyloid (25–35) treatment in mouse models. In 1-methyl-4-phenyl-1,2,3,6-tetrahydropyridine (MPTP) and nitropropionic acid–intoxicated mice, which showed symptoms of Parkinson's disease and brain ischemia, respectively, withanolide A restored cognitive and behavioral aspects. An increase in gluta-thione (GSH) biosynthesis, a reduction in neurodegeneration, and a reversal of hypoxia-induced GSH depletion in the hippocampus were observed.
- Wi-N protects brain cells from oxidative, glutamate, and MAA (a phthalate biotoxin) stress by reducing ROS and damage to DNA and mitochondria. Phthalates are a class of industrial chemicals used to soften polyvinyl chlo-ride plastic and as solvents in cosmetics and other consumer products. They are also widely used in agriculture, medicine, and everyday household prod-ucts and are readily absorbed by the human body, where they are converted to toxic metabolites and threaten a variety of tissue functions. In experiments with human cells, Wi-N was found to protect cells from MAA toxicity.

4.7   COGNITIVE DYSFUNCTION

Cognitive dysfunction often results in a variety of neurophysiological abnormalities. Ashwagandha improves auditory-verbal memory, social cognition, and reaction time associated with bipolar disorder and other neuropsychiatric conditions and ameliorates their symptoms. Improved locomotor and cognitive functions during aging have been noted and attributed to modulation of GABAergic activity, α-amino-3-hydroxy-5-methyl-4-isoxazolepropionic acid (AMPA) receptor function, and N-methyl-D-aspartate (NMDA) receptor density.

4.8   ISCHEMIA

Stroke is a leading cause of brain injury and is caused by ischemia when the brain is deprived of oxygen and essential nutrients due to cholesterol buildup blocking the arteries (atherosclerosis). Research shows that Ashwagandha protects cells from ischemia and reperfusion injury, thereby preventing stroke. It reduces oxidative stress, restores vital cellular activity, and improves behavioral deficits. In addition, an aqueous extract of Ashwagandha leaves may prevent neurotoxicity in brain cells by producing proteins that help neurons adapt.

4.9   ALZHEIMER'S DISEASE

Alzheimer's disease is a major age-related neurodegenerative disorder. It is best defined as a progressive loss of both short-term and long-term memory and cognitive function (movement, balance, and behavioral abnormalities) that becomes increasingly severe and has a poor prognosis. Approximately 18 million people worldwide are currently being treated for Alzheimer's disease, and this number is expected to grow to 34 million by 2025.

- Medically, Alzheimer's disease is characterized by the formation of protein plaques in the brain consisting of β-amyloid and tau proteins. The disease not only affects a patient's life expectancy and quality of life but also severely impacts families, social dynamics, and the global economy in terms of managing and treating the disease. Natural medicines are highly valued for the prevention and treatment of Alzheimer's disease. Because Ashwagandha can reverse the cytotoxicity caused by many environmental toxins, many laboratories have evaluated its potential to mitigate the effects of Alzheimer's disease. Research data from many laboratories have provided evidence that Ashwagandha protects brain cells from endogenous toxins such as neurotoxic peptides, including β-amyloid, which is found in the brains of Alzheimer's disease and Down syndrome patients. It also improves the symptoms of the human immunodeficiency virus (HIV)–associated dementia, which causes a wide range of neurological complications, including cognitive, behavioral, and motor abnormalities. Because HIV is a human-specific virus, animal models of HIV infection have not been very successful in providing mechanistic insights into its neuropathology.

However, cultured human cells have been used consistently and success-fully for research; some of the major findings are listed below.

- Ashwagandha withanolides (specifically withanolide A and withanoside IV) and withanamides prevent neuronal death caused by amyloid protein plaques. The compounds also protect the density, area, and length of spines on neuron dendrites, which are projections from the cell that receive signals from other neurons. Withanoside A primarily affects neuron axons, which are extensions of cells that send signals to other neurons. Withanoside IV affects dendrite growth, significantly improving memory function and neu-roprotection. Studies have shown remarkable increases in axon density at the cellular level, leading to improvements in object recognition and mem-ory in animal models.

- Reduced synthesis of a neurotransmitter called acetylcholine and loss of neurons that use acetylcholine play a critical role in Alzheimer's disease. Herbal formulations containing Ashwagandha and various withanolides can inhibit the breakdown of acetylcholine by the enzyme acetylcholin-esterase, which is a widely accepted treatment for Alzheimer's disease. Bioinformatics and computational studies have shown that withanolide A binds tightly to the active sites of the human acetylcholinesterase enzyme and inhibits its activity. Cholinesterase inhibitors (donepezil, rivastigmine, and galantamine) have been approved to improve memory and behavior but do not appear to stop the progression of Alzheimer's disease. Withanolides appear to have better results and less toxicity.

- Mice treated with Ashwagandha root extract show clearance of β-amyloid from the brain. Small vessels in the brain of these mice showed increased levels of low-density lipoprotein receptor-related protein (LRP) and neprily-sin (NEP), an Aβ-degrading protease. These data suggest that Ashwagandha extract may aid in the clearance of Aβ and thus may be valuable in the treat-ment of Alzheimer's disease.

- Ashwagandha derivatives with the amides A and C have been shown to bind to β-amyloid and prevent the formation of tangled β-amyloid protein fibers in nerve cells.

- In an experimental mouse model of Alzheimer's disease, supplementation with Ashwagandha root extract helped remove β-amyloid proteins, improve behavioral deficits, and protect neurons from the toxicity caused by the buildup of these proteins. Ashwagandha has also been shown to help ani-mals recover from the stress of immobilization.

- Exposure of cultured glial cells to lead causes severe toxicity. Supplementation with Ashwagandha extracts caused a remarkable reduction in lead-induced toxicity in glial cells and promoted the growth of new projections from neurons.

- Cultured neurons exposed to β-amyloid show strong toxicity. On the con-trary, Ashwagandha extracts restored and rejuvenated synapses in neurons damaged by β-amyloid toxicity. Ashwagandha-treated cells also showed improved spine density, area, length, and number, which are severely reduced by amyloid treatment.

- Ashwagandha withanamides prevent the formation of β-amyloid fibrils and protect cells from the toxic effects of β-amyloid.
- Withanolide A has been shown to modulate several targets associated with the processing of the β-amyloid precursor protein. For example, it has been shown to downregulate beta-secretase 1 (BACE1), an enzyme that helps cells produce β-amyloid from its precursor protein. It also upregulates an enzyme (A disintegrin and metalloprotease 10 (ADAM10)) that is involved in processing the precursor protein.
- In mouse models of Alzheimer's disease, Ashwagandha extracts caused clearance of β-amyloid proteins through the activation of liver enzymes and reversed impairments in spatial learning and working memory. Clearance of β-amyloid peptides in the brain, increased levels of liver low-density LRP, and β-amyloid-degrading protease NEP were observed. Liver LRP mediates the endocytosis of plasma β-amyloid peptides, which are then cleared by NEP and other proteases present in the liver (Figure 4.5).
- High-resolution mass spectrometry techniques show that withanamide crosses the blood–brain barrier in mice when injected into the abdomen. This suggests that the ingestion of the extract may have similar results as it readily crosses cell membranes.
- Using cells differentiated from neural progenitor cells in the human fetal brain, researchers have demonstrated the effect of the HIV-1 protein called transactivator of transcription (Tat) on their proliferative and neurogenic properties. The neurotoxic effects of Tat have also been studied in mature

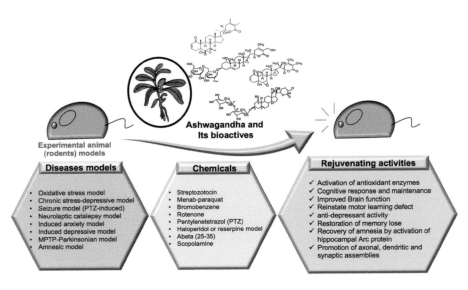

FIGURE 4.5 Pictorial representation of Ashwagandha bioactivities validated by laboratory studies in animal disease models (shown in blue frame) using a variety of chemically induced stresses/diseases (shown in gray frame). Ashwagandha effects that were confirmed in these studies are shown in colored frames (Wadhwa et al., 2017).

neurons differentiated from these cells. Studies using pure cultures of astrocytes and/or neurons differentiated from these cells provide relevant cellular and molecular insights into astrocyte dysfunction and indirect neurotoxicity. It was found that the proliferative and neurogenic abilities of these cells are enhanced upon treatment with Ashwagandha extract and pure withanolide Wi-N.

4.10 PARKINSON'S DISEASE

Parkinson's disease is a neurodegenerative disease caused by the loss of neurons that produce dopamine, a neurotransmitter important for feelings of pleasure and motivation. Parkinson's disease is characterized by muscle rigidity, tremors, motor dysfunction, postural instability, senile movements/speech/posture, and weakness and slowness of movements (called bradykinesia). At the molecular level, the disease is characterized by the loss of dopaminergic neurons in the substantia nigra region of the brain, the formation of Lewy bodies (abnormal deposits of alpha-synuclein (α-Syn) protein), and high levels of oxidative stress. Experimental induction of Parkinson's disease in mice is achieved by exposure to maneb (MB) and paraquat (PQ) and other environmental toxins that induce selective damage to dopaminergic neurons.

- In mouse models of Parkinson's disease, Ashwagandha showed neuroprotective effects by increasing levels of dopamine and its metabolites and normalizing the expression of oxidative stress markers in the brain. These mice showed improved motor function and higher antioxidant levels in the brain, along with reduced oxidative stress and increased levels of neurotransmitters, including dopamine. Consumption of Ashwagandha extract (100 mg/kg body weight) for 8–9 weeks reduced the expression of markers of inflammation and astroglial activation (which occurs in response to cell damage) in these mouse models.
- In a rat model of 6-hydroxydopamine-induced Parkinson's disease, Ashwagandha treatment provided neuroprotective effects against neuronal injury caused by oxidative agents and free radicals. It also caused a reduction in lipid peroxidation, GSH content, activities of GSH S-transferase, GSH reductase, GSH peroxidase, SOD and catalase, catecholamine content, dopaminergic D2 receptor binding, and tyrosine hydroxylase. Reversal of neurobehavioral deficits was observed.
- In another mouse model of Parkinson's disease using MPTP-induced parkinsonism, Ashwagandha supplementation was shown to improve antioxidant and catecholamine levels, ameliorating animal behavior and physical abnormalities such as posture, muscle rigidity, and tremors. Ashwagandha extract at the dose of 100 mg/kg body weight for 7 days helped to rescue from oxidative damage and restore memory loss in Parkinson's mouse models. It significantly induced the levels of SOD, catalase, and malondialdehyde, resulting in reduced levels of GSH and GSH peroxidase in the brain of Parkinson's mice.

- In Parkinson's disease model using rotenone to induce oxidative damage, mice showed an increase in biological markers of stress, including the ROS malondialdehyde (MDA), hydroperoxides (HP), and nitric oxide (NO) in the brain. Inefficient antioxidant defense mechanisms, including reduced levels of GSH (an antioxidant that protects cellular components from ROS), low levels of antioxidant enzymes, and high levels of mitochondrial dysfunction were detected. However, feeding the animals Ashwagandha extract (400 mg/kg body weight) for 4 weeks normalized the levels of oxidative stress markers and restored antioxidant levels.
- One study showed that feeding Ashwagandha extract (100 mg/kg body weight) to mice for 7–28 days increased levels of dopamine and its metabolites and normalized levels of oxidative stress markers in the brain of a mouse model of Parkinson's disease.
- In a model of Parkinson's disease in the fruit fly (*Drosophila melanogaster*), which shows abnormalities in motor response and mitochondrial function, feeding Ashwagandha extract improved motor function and suppressed oxidative stress and mitochondrial dysfunction, resulting in increased lifespan.
- In a cell culture model using cells derived from the human brain, treatment with Ashwagandha prevented cell death caused by the hyperactivation of inflammation.
- In Ayurveda, Ashwagandha is considered to be the most important natural medicine for the treatment of oxidative damage and physiological abnormalities in Parkinson's disease.

4.11 AMNESIA

Amnesia is a neurodegenerative disorder caused by brain damage or psychological trauma that results in memory loss. Traditional home medicine reports that Ashwagandha also treats amnesia. In the laboratory, scopolamine hydrobromide (a plant alkaloid derivative), which induces memory loss and mimics aging and dementia, is used to understand the disease at the animal and cellular levels and to screen anti-amnesia drugs. The scopolamine hydrobromide–induced amnesic mouse model is one of the most widely accepted pharmacological animal models of memory dysfunction. Scopolamine hydrobromide has been shown to be a potent acetylcholine receptor antagonist that inhibits central cholinergic neuronal activity. Rotenone is another neurotoxic compound that causes oxidative stress and mimics the memory and cognitive impairment associated with Parkinson's disease. Representative reports of laboratory studies on the effect of Ashwagandha on amnesia are listed below:

- In a mouse model of amnesia, Ashwagandha leaf extract rich in Wi-N and purified Wi-N improved amnesia symptoms and cognitive response. The extract and compound were shown to achieve these effects by inducing specific proteins called brain-derived neurotrophic factor (BDNF). Scopolamine-treated mice showed remarkable recovery in memory and behavioral parameters when treated with Ashwagandha.

- The beneficial effects of Ashwagandha leaf extract in a mouse model of dementia involve the upregulation of activity-regulated cytoskeleton-associated protein, which plays a critical role in learning and memory. A study showed that the plant metabolites anaferine, β-sitosterol, Wi-A, withanolide A, withanolide B, and withanolide D inhibit receptors critical for signaling between neurons and their adaptability. This suggests that Ashwagandha may have beneficial effects in the treatment of neurodegenerative diseases.
- In cultured cell assays, Ashwagandha extracts rich in Wi-N or purified Wi-N protected brain-derived cells from oxidative and DNA damage. DNA damage induced in brain-derived cells by scopolamine or H_2O_2 was inhibited by Ashwagandha extract or its purified Wi-N component. Both also protect cells against increased ROS, mitochondrial and DNA damage, and premature aging in cultured human cells treated with the industrial metabolite MAA. In addition, cell defense pathways involving antioxidant expression and protein turnover are activated by treatment with Ashwagandha extract or Wi-N.
- Hypoxia (lack of oxygen)–induced models of memory impairment mimic the oxidative damage of memory disorders. Oxygen deprivation at high altitudes causes oxidative stress, degenerates neurons, and impairs memory function. In experimental rat models of this phenomenon, called hypobaric hypoxia, Ashwagandha extracts with potent antioxidant potential were able to reduce stress and restore memory. Crude extracts of Ashwagandha root reduced levels of nitric oxide, corticosterone, and ROS in the hippocampal region of the brain. Withanolide A increased antioxidant levels and reduced overall oxidative stress in hypoxic rats.

4.12 HUNTINGTON'S DISEASE

HD is a fatal neurodegenerative disorder. It is an autosomal dominant neurodegenerative disorder caused by mutation in the huntingtin gene and protein, which is rich in glutamine. Patients with HD have cognitive, motor, and psychiatric disorders. The disease is characterized by the loss of neurons (primarily in striatal and cortical regions of the brain), resulting in abnormalities in muscle coordination, cognition, and behavioral responses.

In Ayurveda, Ashwagandha is believed to be beneficial for individuals with HD. Experimental mouse models of HD are induced by 3-nitro propionic acid, which causes neurophysiological abnormalities, including biochemical, behavioral, and mitochondrial dysfunction, similar to those seen in human patients. Laboratory studies have demonstrated the benefits of Ashwagandha in mouse models of HD. Administration of Ashwagandha extracts to these mice increased levels of antioxidant enzymes and restored energy storage in a dose-dependent manner. It also caused remarkable improvements in cognitive (tested by the Morris water maze test and elevated plus maze test) and motor functions (tested by impairment of muscle activity as observed in the rotarod and limb withdrawal test) in HD mice. Ashwagandha-treated mice showed reduced oxidative stress, restored antioxidants, and increased activity of an enzyme required for proper neuronal function.

4.13   AMYOTROPHIC LATERAL SCLEROSIS

Amyotrophic lateral sclerosis (ALS) is a progressive disease that causes the degeneration of nerve cells, primarily motor neurons that control voluntary muscles. It differs from Alzheimer's disease, Parkinson's disease, and HD in that it involves the spinal cord and brain. ALS is caused by a progressive breakdown of the protective sheath that surrounds nerve cells, called the myelin sheath. The majority of people diagnosed with ALS die of respiratory failure within 3–5 years of the onset of symptoms; less than 10% of patients survive for 10 years or more. Like several other neurodegenerative and cognitive diseases, ALS is characterized by the loss of mitochondrial function and increased levels of toxic proteins in the brain.

Despite continued efforts over the past several decades, there are no effective therapies for ALS. This is partly because the disease is caused by multiple factors, making it difficult to treat with a single drug that targets a specific factor, pathway, or mechanism. Major changes reported in ALS tissues include large-scale structural breakdown in regions of the brain (frontal and anterior temporal lobes) and microscopic changes in cells. Insoluble forms of tau, the protein implicated in Alzheimer's disease, are often found in ALS tissue.

ALS is often complicated by spinal cord injury, which inhibits the flow of sensory, motor, and reflex information between the body and the brain. The changes that are associated with spinal cord injury can include the degeneration of axons, loss of neurons and glial cells, and invasion of peripheral immune cells. Several model systems have been established to study spinal cord injury. Ashwagandha has been reported to benefit ALS in the following ways

- Oral administration of withanoside IV 1 hour after spinal cord injury induces axon growth in the spinal cord and helps restore motor function in the hind limbs.
- Ashwagandha promotes neuronal differentiation, regeneration, and adaptability.
- Ashwagandha caused the activation of antioxidant defense mechanisms and function of acetylcholine receptors. It also inhibited the enzyme that breaks down acetylcholine.
- In ALS, misfolded proteins cause stress and increase oxidative damage in certain parts of the cell, including mitochondria, ER, DNA, proteins, and lipids. These changes have been linked to motor neuron death in some models of ALS. Ashwagandha extracts protected against these stresses and improved ALS symptoms.
- In a mouse model of chronic stress, Ashwagandha root extracts or purified components showed anti-stress effects by acting as potent antioxidants.
- In one study, Wi-A significantly improved disease pathology, including reducing glial cell activation and improving motor performance in a variety of tests in mouse models of the disease. It also modestly increased the median survival time of the mice.
- Wi-A-treated mice showed increased levels of stress regulatory proteins [heat shock protein 70 (HSP70) and HSP25)], which contribute to overall neuroprotection.

- Wi-A activates the Keap1/Nrf2 pathway, an important regulator of antioxidants in the body, and has protective or therapeutic effects through these antioxidant and anti-inflammatory properties. It also reduces gliosis-dependent inflammation in experimental mouse models.
- Wi-A inhibits high-mobility group box 1 (HMGB1) protein, which is elevated in patients with ALS.
- Wi-A binds to the intermediate filament proteins vimentin, peripherin, and glial acidic fibrillary protein (GFAP) on astrocytes, which are elevated in ALS.
- Wi-A, withanolide A, withanoside IV, Wi-N, and withanamides are the biologically active compounds that have been shown to be primarily responsible for the reported neuroprotective activities of Ashwagandha extracts.

4.14 TARDIVE DYSKINESIA

Tardive dyskinesia is a syndrome characterized by repetitive involuntary movements, usually involving the mouth, face, tongue, limbs, and trunk muscles. Tardive dyskinesia is an important side effect of long-term treatment with antipsychotic drugs. It can be induced by treatment with neuroleptic haloperidol in experimental animal models. Ashwagandha extracts, rich in withanolides, have been reported to have beneficial effects on the symptoms of the disease. In mouse models, Ashwagandha extract inhibited involuntary mouth or face movements, chewing movements, tongue protrusion, and shaking of the mouth or cheek muscles (called buccal tremor).

4.15 EPILEPSY

Epilepsy is a chronic, multi-symptom disorder characterized by recurrent seizures. It is mainly caused by an imbalance between stimulatory and inhibitory neurons, in which the neurotransmitters glutamate and GABA play an important role. Ashwagandha extract has antioxidant effects, inhibiting toxic overactivation of neurons and oxidative damage in the brain. Extracts also help prevent seizures in pentylenetetrazol-induced models of epilepsy by modulating the GABA-based system. Extract and withanolide A both improve spatial memory deficits by enhancing antioxidant systems and restoring glutamate receptors in temporal lobe epilepsy. In a rodent model of temporal lobe epilepsy, Ashwagandha extract restored AMPA receptor function. In an experimental mouse model of epilepsy, Ashwagandha extract and withanolide A showed neuroprotective activity and were able to reverse spatial memory loss. The primary mechanism of action of these ingredients was the reduction of oxidative stress, thereby preventing neurodegeneration and inhibiting blocked signaling between neurons. Epileptic rodents have significant degeneration of hippocampal neurons and increased oxidative damage, as shown by increased levels of SOD and catalase enzyme activities. These animals are also deficient in hippocampus-dependent spatial memory. Administration of either Ashwagandha root extract or withanolide A alone significantly attenuated the increased gene expression and enzyme activity, restoring them to near-normal levels. Treatment with the extract also reduced increased lipid peroxidation in rat models of epilepsy. The antioxidant activities of the extract help rescue neuronal death in the hippocampus and improve memory.

4.16   BIPOLAR DISORDER

Bipolar disorder is a mood disorder. It is often lifelong, with episodes of mania and depression interspersed with periods of remission. Patients have cognitive impairment and deficits in attention, concentration, memory, and executive function, even during periods when they are relatively well. This can severely interfere with daily activities. Symptoms often include maladaptive behaviors, illicit substance abuse, poor mental judgment, reckless spending and impulsivity, and depressive or manic episodes. Medications for bipolar disorder include lithium, anticonvulsants (such as valproate, aripiprazole, lamotrigine, ziprasidone, and carbamazepine), and antipsychotics (such as olanzapine, quetiapine, risperidone, asenapine, paliperidone, and lurasidone). People with mania have low levels of neurotrophin (BDNF) and high levels of glutamate, an excitatory neurotransmitter in the brain, and they often develop hypothyroidism in response to lithium treatment. Ashwagandha extracts have been tested for the treatment of thyroid-induced cognitive dysfunction in people with bipolar disorder.

- Animal studies have shown that the bioactive constituents of Ashwagandha, namely steroidal lactones such as glycowithanolides, sitoindosides, and Wi-A, have potent antioxidant, neuroprotective, and memory-enhancing properties in the brain. A review of eight markers of oxidative stress in bipolar disorder (SOD, catalase, GSH peroxidase, protein carbonyl, 3-nitro-tyrosine, lipid peroxidation, nitric oxide, and RNA/DNA damage) in 971 patients with bipolar disorder and 886 controls showed that patients with bipolar disorder have increased DNA/RNA damage, nitric oxide, and especially lipid peroxidation compared to controls.
- In a comprehensive review of rodent models of brain oxidative stress (including prolonged swimming, sleep deprivation, and chemical and physical restraint stress), pretreatment of mice with Ashwagandha extracts normalized levels of antioxidant enzymes (GSH peroxidase, SOD, and catalase) and reduced levels of the antioxidant GSH.
- Ashwagandha reduces lipid peroxidation products (malondialdehyde and thiobarbituric acid reactive substances) that cause neuronal dysfunction and damage in certain brain regions, namely the hippocampus, striatum, and forebrain.
- In an animal model of restraint stress, in which nitric oxide levels caused a marked increase in neuronal dysfunction, Ashwagandha pretreatment significantly reduced elevated nitric oxide levels. Chronic administration of Ashwagandha extracts significantly reduced lipid peroxidation and restored GSH, SOD, and catalase levels in a rat brain model of dyskinesia and cognitive dysfunction.
- In a rat stress model, feeding the animals with Ashwagandha extract significantly improved their poor memory retention. In an immobilization stress test, Ashwagandha extract reduced damage to hippocampal neurons by nearly 80%.

- In a rat model of streptozotocin-induced behavioral cognitive deficits characterized by increased oxidative stress and cholinergic neuronal dysfunction, the group fed with Ashwagandha extract showed recovery of choline acetyltransferase activity and the ability to produce the neurotransmitter acetylcholine.
- Treatment of mice with Ashwagandha extracts for 3 weeks improved their cognitive deficits, restored antioxidant status, and improved signal transmission between neurons.
- Glutamate excitotoxicity has been reported when bipolar patients experience mania, and unchecked glutamate excitotoxicity can lead to loss of neuronal function (resulting in cognitive problems) as well as neuronal and glial cell death. Ashwagandha aqueous extract not only improved glutamate excitotoxicity in cultured rat glioma and human neuroblastoma cells but also significantly reduced protein markers of neuronal viability (such as HSP70) while inducing the expression of proteins that enhance neural plasticity, learning, and memory [such as neural cell adhesion molecule (NCAM)].
- Ashwagandha extracts have demonstrated anti-stress, anti-anxiety, anti-inflammatory, cortisol-lowering, and cytokine and monoamine-modulating properties in animal and human studies. Thus, Ashwagandha extracts show promise as a potential adjunct treatment for cognitive impairment and mood swings in people with bipolar disorder.
- A randomized clinical trial tested aqueous Ashwagandha extracts in 60 patients with bipolar disorder for 8 weeks. Patients were treated with 250 mg of extract (containing a minimum of 8% withanolides, a maximum of 2% Wi-A, and 32% oligosaccharides) once daily for the first week and 250 mg twice daily for the remainder of the study. Patients then underwent computerized neuropsychological testing to assess their cognition. Three cognitive tasks (measures of auditory-verbal working memory, reaction time, and social cognition) improved significantly in patients treated with Ashwagandha extract. There were no adverse effects on physical activity or weight gain. Although bipolar patients have relatively higher rates of hypothyroidism, Ashwagandha extracts improved thyroid measures and subclinical hypothyroidism.

4.17 NEUROINFLAMMATION

In animal models of inflammation or arthritis, Ashwagandha extracts have shown anti-inflammatory activity. This activity includes decreased levels of some inflammatory markers (acute phase reactants, prostaglandin synthesis, and α-2 macroglobulin). Ashwagandha extract blocked the nuclear factor kappa B (NF-kB) inflammatory signaling pathway in cells from both healthy individuals and patients with rheumatoid arthritis, resulting in suppressed production of several pro-inflammatory signaling molecules called cytokines. Withanolides also strongly block COX-2 enzyme activity, which is closely related to the efficacy of anti-inflammatory drugs.

4.18   SCHIZOPHRENIA AND ANXIETY

Schizophrenia is a neurological disorder involving abnormal metabolism and function of neurotransmitters in the brain, including dopamine, glutamate, GABA, acetylcholine, and serotonin. Ashwagandha has been shown to enhance the function of neurons that signal through the neurotransmitters dopamine, glutamate, and acetylcholine, thus protecting the neurons. The Positive and Negative Syndrome Scale is a medical scale of behavioral tests used to measure symptom severity in patients with schizophrenia. It is considered the gold standard test for antipsychotic behavioral disorders and is used for disease diagnosis, treatment, and prognosis. Ashwagandha has been shown to reduce the symptoms of schizophrenia and alleviate the effects of associated neurological abnormalities, including the following results.

- In double-blind, placebo-controlled trials in patients with schizophrenia and anxiety disorders, Ashwagandha extract (300–500 mg) produced moderate to excellent symptom improvement within 2 weeks. In addition, 72% of patients showed improvement and continued to take the extract for up to 18 months. Patients reported a satisfactory reduction in anxiety symptoms with no adverse effects.
- In another double-blind, randomized study of patients with chronic stress or mild to severe anxiety, Ashwagandha significantly improved stress tolerance, recovery from anxiety, and self-rated quality of life, with no adverse symptoms. These benefits were seen within 2 months, suggesting the health safety of Ashwagandha.
- The effects of Ashwagandha extract were studied in a rat model of ethanol withdrawal, which causes anxiety and depression. In this test, rats were given access to ethanol through a liquid diet for 15 days. On day 16, the animals were placed on an ethanol-free liquid diet and assessed for anxiety and depression. Administration of Ashwagandha extract reduced anxiety in the rats. This effect was attributed to the plant's GABA-mimicking properties.
- Obsessive-compulsive disorder (OCD) is an anxiety-related mental disorder. It is characterized by persistent depression and is usually treated with antidepressants that inhibit serotonin. Treatment of a mouse model of OCD with Ashwagandha extract showed that it was as effective as the standard anti-OCD drug fluoxetine.
- Benzo[a]pyrene (B[a]P), a prototype polycyclic aromatic hydrocarbon, is known to cause neurotoxicity and behavioral alterations. In a zebrafish model of B[a]P-induced behavioral changes, an aqueous leaf extract of Ashwagandha was shown to have anxiolytic effects and is therefore recommended for the treatment of anxiety symptoms.
- Researchers have studied the effects of Ashwagandha extracts on neuroplasticity (the brain's ability to synthesize and reorganize synaptic and neuronal connections in response to any environmental stimulus or injury) and neuroregeneration (a process that leads to the repair of damaged neurons or connections, resulting in the recovery of neuronal function) in cell culture and animal models. In a human neuroblastoma cell line, Ashwagandha

extract caused a dose-dependent increase in the percentage of neuronal population with significant neurite outgrowth, with clear upregulation of proteins involved in synaptic and neuronal growth. Withanolide A, withanoside IV, and withanoside VI were identified as the active components responsible for this activity. These withanolides also induced axon growth and increased synaptic density even in the presence of β-amyloid protein in both cell culture and animal models of Alzheimer's disease. In addition, oral withanoside IV for 21 days induces axon growth in the spinal cord and restores motor function in the hind limbs.

- Withanoside IV improved memory in a mouse model of Alzheimer's disease. Its major metabolite, sominone, was shown to have significant regenerative potential. It caused the reconstruction of neuronal connections and improved memory in mice. Similar effects of withanoside IV were observed in injured neurons, where it enhanced synaptogenesis and neurite outgrowth in the brain.
- In a study conducted on post-myocardial infarction patients, Ashwagandha extract, administered in the form of an herbal cocktail, was able to improve their quality of life, reduce cholesterol and triglyceride levels, and increase high-density lipoprotein cholesterol very effectively.
- Consistent with the fact that Ashwagandha supplements induce relaxation and calmness in the body, many reports suggest the use of Ashwagandha to treat neuropsychiatric conditions, including anxiety and depression.
- Ashwagandha-derived bioactive glycowithanolides were able to reduce the levels of the anxiety marker tribulin in the rat brain.
- Oral administration of Ashwagandha alleviates anxiety induced by ethanol withdrawal in ethanol-dependent rats. Additional beneficial behavioral and physiological effects of Ashwagandha were observed in these rats, suggesting that Ashwagandha could be used to treat anxiety associated with ethanol withdrawal.
- The anxiolytic effects of Ashwagandha extracts are comparable to the standard anti-anxiety drug diazepam as well as several commercially available antipsychotics, including fluoxetine, gabapentin, citalopram, clozapine, risperidone, and venlafaxine.
- The anti-anxiety activity of Ashwagandha has also been demonstrated in a behavioral comparison. In this randomized comparative trial, individuals with moderate to severe anxiety were treated with either a naturopathic intervention (consisting of dietary strategies, relaxation, and Ashwagandha supplementation) or a standard psychotherapy intervention (consisting of psychotherapy, relaxation, and placebo medication) for 12 weeks. Although both approaches significantly reduced patients' anxiety, the Ashwagandha group reported further reductions in anxiety compared to the psychotherapy group.
- Ashwagandha has also been found to reduce plasma corticosterone levels and improve chronic stress-induced adrenal and spleen enlargement in rats.
- Ashwagandha supplements improved anxiety caused by OCD in mouse models.

- Antidepressant effects of Ashwagandha have been shown in a variety of experimental models, with antidepressant activity comparable to the antidepressant drug imipramine.
- Ashwagandha is widely accepted as a mood stabilizer in clinical psychiatric conditions and is used to alleviate depression. This effect is mediated by the activation of two different systems in the body: adrenergic systems, which rely on signaling by adrenaline-based neurotransmitters, and serotonergic systems, which rely on signaling by serotonin-based neurotransmitters. Ashwagandha treatment also reduced the risk of behavioral and neural side effects of drugs called antipsychotics, such as haloperidol, which is used to treat schizophrenia.
- In a mouse model of depression, an Ashwagandha-containing herbal formulation was found to significantly inhibit despair, moderate anti-reserpine activity and sedation and caused remarkable improvement in chronic fatigue syndrome. With such improved behavioral, psychological, and biochemical activities, Ashwagandha supplements are suggested to have potent antidepressant activity.
- Two randomized clinical trials (one for 6 weeks and the other for 12 weeks) showed anxiety-reducing activity of Ashwagandha extracts in patients with anxiety disorders. In an Ayurvedic clinic, a randomized clinical trial treated stressed individuals with Ashwagandha extracts for 2 months. This study demonstrated the efficacy of Ashwagandha in relieving stress symptoms and reducing elevated levels of the stress hormone cortisol and the inflammatory marker c-reactive protein. Ashwagandha extracts, combined with other herbal extracts, have shown efficacy in arthritic and other pain measures, with patients reporting only mild side effects. A recent 8-week randomized clinical trial of Ashwagandha for weight management in stressed adults showed positive results, including weight loss, improved stress scores, and reduced cortisol levels compared to a group that did not receive Ashwagandha.

4.19 CATALEPSY

Catalepsy is a neurological disorder in which a person experiences seizures with loss of consciousness and an immobilized, rigid body state. Catalepsy is often associated with hysteria and other complex cerebellar disorders. In animal model studies, Ashwagandha protected against catalepsy induced by treatment with the antipsychotic drugs haloperidol or reserpine. In the haloperidol-induced catalepsy mouse model, treatments with Ashwagandha derivatives restore postural problems, increase antioxidant potential, and reduce neurological abnormalities and oxidative stress.

4.20 INSOMNIA

Good sleep is closely linked to rejuvenation, restoring the body's functional resources and neutralizing toxins. On the contrary, lack of sleep causes low energy, exhausts the body, and severely affects work efficiency. Insomnia is a sleep disorder in which difficulty falling asleep or staying asleep at night affects quality of life, resulting in daytime sleepiness, low energy, irritability, and depressed mood. It is one of the most common neuropsychiatric disorders, with an estimated incidence of 10%–15% in the general population and 30%–60% in the elderly. Insomnia is often associated with anxiety, stress, fatigue, anger, worry, grief, mania, bipolar disorder, and trauma. Insomnia also results in significant economic losses to society due to traffic accidents, lost work productivity, and clinical treatment costs. Sleep abnormalities are believed to increase the risk of serious neurodegenerative diseases, including Alzheimer's disease, Parkinson's disease, dementia, and ALS.

- Most commercially available drugs used to treat insomnia are based on benzodiazepines, melatonin modulators, or antihistamines. These drugs are often associated with major or minor side effects such as addiction and withdrawal symptoms. On the contrary, Ashwagandha has been reported to induce physical calm and relaxation and to alleviate insomnia. These effects have been associated with a reduced risk of neuronal degeneration. In Ayurveda, Ashwagandha is used to promote healthy sleep – in fact, *somnifera* in Latin means "sleep inducer" – by rejuvenating the body and alleviating stress-related fatigue. As an adaptogen, Ashwagandha regulates hormone secretion by the adrenal glands and helps the body cope with stress. Research and anecdotal evidence show that Ashwagandha can improve insomnia, with effects seen as early as 5–7 days after treatment. In comparison, the effects on depression and anxiety may take a few weeks. Research provides many lines of evidence for Ashwagandha's anti-insomnia activity and possible mechanisms of action.
- Ashwagandha-derived alkaloids or their combination with diazepam have been shown to reverse sleep loss in mouse sleep models. They improved catalase, activated GABAergic signaling, and caused remarkable reductions in lipid peroxidation and nitrite levels.
- Healthy human volunteers using Ashwagandha reported an improvement in sleep quality.
- Overproduction of the stress hormone cortisol is one cause of insomnia. In a normal circadian clock, cortisol naturally decreases toward evening in preparation for sleep. Conditions such as stress/depression/anxiety increase and maintain cortisol levels, thereby interfering with sleep. In numerous independent research reports, Ashwagandha has been shown to limit cortisol production.
- GABA is a neurotransmitter that facilitates communication between brain cells and determines relaxed and stressed states. The function of GABA depends on the proper response of GABA receptors in brain cells. Many drugs interact with GABA and GABA receptors in the brain to alter their function, resulting in effects such as relaxation, pain relief, stress and anxiety reduction, lowered blood pressure, and improved sleep. Ashwagandha may mimic GABA to positively affect the neuronal receptors responsible for receiving GABA and reduce neuronal excitability, resulting in a relaxed state of mind.

- Many environmental toxins affect the brain, which has natural detoxification mechanisms to release toxins through drainage systems during sleep. Poor sleep results in inadequate removal of toxins. Ashwagandha may induce an antioxidant effect in the brain, protecting against heavy metal damage and aiding in detoxification.
- Hypoglycemia is a condition of low blood sugar levels that makes it difficult for the body to function properly. It is often associated with diabetes. Nocturnal hypoglycemia is low blood sugar at night and is also common in people with diabetes. It causes dizziness, lightheadedness, and blurred vision and is closely associated with insomnia. The drop in blood glucose levels causes the release of glucose-regulating hormones that stimulate the desire to eat. During nocturnal hypoglycemia, a patient perceives a signal to wake up and eat, which disrupts sleep and reduces sleep quality. Eating before bed helps stabilize blood sugar levels and prevents the sudden drop that signals the adrenal glands to release adrenaline and cortisol, which disrupts sleep patterns. Several studies show that Ashwagandha is beneficial for nocturnal hypoglycemia–related insomnia. It significantly reduces stress and insomnia and helps regulate blood glucose to normal levels, reducing stress and mood swings and supporting healthy body weight management (Figure 4.6).

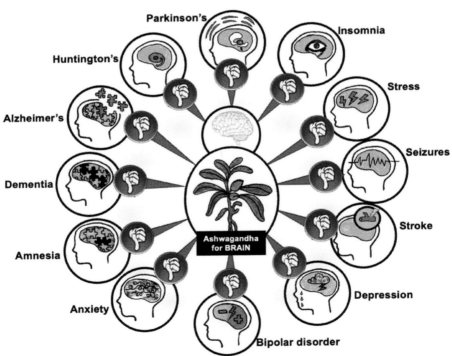

FIGURE 4.6 Pictorial representation of the bioactivities of Ashwagandha for brain disorders.

- Somnogenic ingredient – Although Ayurveda recommends Ashwagandha root or whole plant extract for good sleep, its active sleep-inducing components remain unidentified. In a study, the effect of different components of Ashwagandha leaf on sleep regulation was investigated by feeding them to mice. The results showed that the alcohol extract of Ashwagandha leaf containing active withanolides did not induce sleep in mice. However, water extract of Ashwagandha leaf containing TEG induced significant non-rapid eye movement sleep with smaller changes in rapid eye movement sleep. The researchers validated this finding by treating mice with pure TEG, suggesting that it is an active sleep-inducing component.
- Sleep-deprived mice fed Ashwagandha aqueous extract show reduced anxiety-like behavior along with reduced expression of pro-inflammatory cytokines (TNFα, IL-1β, and IL-6).
- Another study reported the beneficial role of Ashwagandha in preventing memory impairment in rats subjected to short-term sleep deprivation. Feeding rats with an aqueous extract of Ashwagandha for 15 days before sleep deprivation prevented memory loss. In several other studies, Ashwagandha has been shown to help ameliorate stress-induced cognitive impairment by restoring the expression of proteins that help synapses adapt.

4.21 AGING BRAIN AND MEMORY DEFICITS

Like other organs, the brain undergoes anatomical and physiological changes during aging, including reduced volume, expansion of the ventricular system, reduced number of synapses and synaptic spines, and reduced length of myelinated axons. These changes affect the brain's ability to adapt and affect its networks, leading to age-related memory deficits. Although brain aging leads to delayed recall of information and greater difficulty in learning new information, not all types of memory are affected equally in this process. Aging affects how we remember specific events and experiences, known as episodic memory. However, aging does not seem to significantly affect the ability to recall words, concepts, or numbers, called semantic memory, although older people often fail to remember specific details. Aged people also show difficulty in manipulating, reorganizing, and integrating the contents of working memory. Ashwagandha has been shown to be a powerful memory enhancer.

- In animal models of memory impairment, Ashwagandha extracts have shown tremendous potential to restore memory function. It modulates neurotransmitters, rescues oxidative damage, enhances neural plasticity, and regenerates damaged neurons and synapses.
- Impaired signaling of brain neurons via the neurotransmitter acetylcholine (called cholinergic neurons) due to neuron degeneration or problems with receptor signaling is important in memory decline. Reduced function of cholinergic neurons is central to aging and to the memory deficits associated with Alzheimer's disease. Therefore, agents that stimulate the cholinergic system are important for recovery. Ashwagandha extracts increase acetylcholine receptor binding and acetylcholinesterase activity (an enzyme

that breaks down acetylcholine, an important part of signaling) and attenuate amnesia caused by acetylcholine receptor blockade in experimental rats.

- Ashwagandha root extract and its components Wi-A and withanolide A were seen to modulate the brain's inhibitory GABA receptors, causing an increase in the level of NMDA receptors that increase signaling (called NMDA receptors) and reverse memory loss.

- Hippocampal induction of long-term potentiation is the major cellular mechanism of memory. It requires the activation of NMDA receptors by glycine. Ashwagandha extract has been reported to act as a glycine mimetic, resulting in NMDA receptor–mediated neurotransmission and memory enhancement.

- Repair of damaged neuronal networks, including regeneration of dendrites and axons and reconstruction of synaptic connections, is necessary to reverse memory loss. Processes such as the growth of new neurons and synapses strengthen neuronal networks in healthy individuals and are associated with improved memory function. Various extracts of Ashwagandha have been shown to regenerate damaged neurons in models of memory impairment and to enhance existing networks in healthy individuals.

- Administration of Ashwagandha crude root extract and its active constituents (withanolide A, withanoside IV, withanoside VI, and sominone) increases axon growth and reforms synapses in cell culture models. These phytochemicals also have regenerative potential in damaged cortical neurons and improve spatial and recognition memory in mouse models of Alzheimer's disease. Sominone, the active derivative of withanoside VI, stimulates the growth of neuronal projections and enhances memory even in normal mice.

- Oral administration of Ashwagandha extract stabilized mitochondrial functions and prevented oxidative damage in the hypothalamus of diabetic rats. Withanolide A increased GSH biosynthesis in neuronal cells by upregulating γ-glutamyl cysteinyl ligase activity.

- Ashwagandha extract prevented downregulation of neuronal (NF-H, MAP2, PSD-95, GAP-43, BDNF) and glial cell (GFAP) markers and upregulation of DNA damage and oxidative stress in brain-derived cells.

- Sominone, the active metabolite of withanoside IV, increases the density of axons and dendrites in the hippocampus of treated animals.

- Another study reported results suggesting that withanolide A predominantly extends axons, while withanosides IV and VI predominantly extend dendrites.

- Ashwagandha extract improved recognition memory and locomotor coordination in obese rats. The extract was shown to cause upregulation of BDNF and its receptor, both of which were reduced in obese mice. These mice had activation of the PI3K/Akt pathway of cell survival and adaptability, supporting that Ashwagandha extracts have neuroprotective effects.

- Ashwagandha treatment suppressed the release of the stress hormone corticosterone and activated the enzyme that makes the neurotransmitter acetylcholine, thereby increasing serotonin levels in the hippocampus of mice.

- In studies of cultured human neuroblastoma and rat glioblastoma cells, treatment with Ashwagandha extracts or its specific constituents could alleviate oxidative stress, promote survival, maintain cell function, and increase proteins that mark cell specialization (differentiation).

As described above, animal models of disease (most commonly rodents due to cost, availability, and ease of use) are used to understand disease and to test new drugs to minimize adverse effects in humans. However, normal and disease mechanisms in rodents often differ from those in humans. Because of these species differences, human cell cultures are used in the laboratory. In cell culture studies, Ashwagandha promotes the growth of neuronal projections (including axons and dendrites), increases synapse density, and is predicted to improve memory. Ashwagandha also has protective effects against β-amyloid-induced dysfunction of astrocytes.

4.22 DIABETES

Blood sugar in the human body is maintained by two pancreatic hormones, insulin and glucagon. Blood glucose levels rise after eating food. In response to these high sugar levels, β cells in the pancreas secrete insulin into the bloodstream. Insulin helps the body use glucose from carbohydrates in food to produce energy immediately or to store excess glucose in the liver for later use. In this way, insulin helps keep blood sugar levels from getting too high, called hyperglycemia, or too low, called hypoglycemia. Glucagon is a hormone secreted by α cells in the pancreas. It helps break down glycogen stored in the liver into glucose. Glucagon and insulin are part of a feedback system that keeps blood glucose levels stable. If our bodies do not produce enough insulin, or if our cells do not respond to insulin, we can develop hyperglycemia or diabetes.

Diabetes is defined as a condition of high blood glucose levels. This condition interferes with several essential bodily functions and greatly affects quality of life. Because the kidneys have a limit to reabsorbing glucose, excess glucose is excreted in the urine, which is called glucosuria. This increases the osmotic pressure of the urine and also prevents the kidney from reabsorbing water, resulting in increased urine production and fluid loss from the body. In addition to insulin and glucagon, many other gastrointestinal hormones are involved in diabetes. Gut microbes play a critical role in regulating the balance of gastrointestinal hormones and have been linked to many chronic diseases, including diabetes and obesity.

Ayurveda describes diabetes as a metabolic disorder resulting in sweet-tasting urine. Food choices, eating habits, and physical and mental exercises are prescribed to prevent and cure diabetes. Several preclinical and clinical studies of Ashwagandha powder have supported its preventive and therapeutic potential for diabetes, including the following:

- Ashwagandha improved diabetic symptoms in a rat model of the disease. It increased the production and release of insulin from pancreatic cells.
- Ashwagandha prevented and cured disorders of glucose homeostasis. It was shown to be most effective in regulating body weight and glucose metabolism in both diabetic and stressed non-diabetic conditions.

- Ashwagandha protected against oxidative stress and other free radical-induced pathologies in pancreatic β cells. In patients with diabetes mellitus, oxidative stress induced by the dysregulation of glucose homeostasis causes chronic inflammation that eventually leads to tissue damage.
- Ashwagandha extracts and their bioactive constituents inhibit the activities of α-amylase and α-glucosidase, enzymes that help break down starch, as well as digestive processes that regulate glucose levels.
- Daily consumption of Ashwagandha (400 mg/kg/day for several weeks) is well tolerated by diabetic or stressed rodents. The estimated minimum daily dose that could alter insulin sensitivity and glucose homeostasis in rodent models is 25 mg/kg/day.
- Glycowithanolides and their derivative aglycones are some of the bioactive constituents of Ashwagandha that have been shown to have anti-diabetic and oxidative stress protective effects.
- Hyperlipidemia, or high triglyceride levels, is a major risk factor for cardiovascular disease, stroke, and type 2 diabetes. It can also eventually lead to dementia such as Alzheimer's disease. Several studies have reported anti-hyperlipidemic and other beneficial effects of Ashwagandha withanolides against altered lipid metabolism in diabetic or hyperlipidemic animals.
- Ashwagandha reduces the activity of HMG-CoA, the enzyme that regulates cholesterol synthesis, in the liver of cholesterol-fed rats.
- Ashwagandha supplementation increased bile acid synthesis and improved the antioxidant status of the animals.
- Diabetic patients show structural and functional abnormalities in the nervous system, including encephalopathy and myelopathy in the central nervous system and peripheral neuropathy in the peripheral nervous system. Several reports have demonstrated antidepressant, anxiolytic, and other beneficial effects of daily consumption of Ashwagandha and its metabolites in various neurological disorders as well as diabetic and stressed states in rodents.
- Consumption of Ashwagandha root powder (3 g/day) has potassium-sparing diuretic effects in mildly diabetic patients maintained on the anti-diabetic drug Daonil (glibenclamide). Ashwagandha root powder supplementation also reduced serum cholesterol and triglyceride levels in patients with mildly elevated cholesterol levels who were not taking any medication. No side effects were reported.
- One study showed a significant reduction in mean total blood cholesterol and blood urea nitrogen levels. Treatment with Ashwagandha extract for 30 days did not significantly affect blood glucose, triglyceride, and cholesterol levels in non-diabetic control subjects. On the contrary, type 2 diabetics showed significant improvement.
- In a study conducted on human subjects, the hypocholesterolemic, diuretic, and hypoglycemic effects of the hydroalcoholic extract of Ashwagandha were evaluated. Increased urine volume and urinary sodium and decreased triglycerides, serum cholesterol, and low-density lipoprotein were observed in the treated subjects.

4.23 SKIN PIGMENTATION

Skin is our largest tissue and is in direct contact with the environment. Skin hygiene is associated with many diseases, some of which are infectious. Therefore, it is extremely important to take care of our skin health. Besides cosmetic factors, the appearance, quality, and color of the skin are important attributes in daily life. Skin color is controlled by a biological process called melanogenesis, in which specialized skin cells produce a pigment called melanin. The amount and type of pigment determines our skin color. Ultraviolet B (UVB) radiation causes darkening of the pigments in the skin (such as melanosis or solar lentigo). This involves the activation of an enzyme called tyrosinase and the production and secretion of immune signaling molecules called cytokines.

Under normal skin conditions, tyrosinase functions in a tightly regulated manner to synthesize melanin in melanosomes and maintain the constitutive level of skin color. The cosmetic industry worldwide has been developing anti-pigmentation agents that could block melanin formation by either degrading tyrosinase or preventing melanin from moving from melanocytes (where it is produced) to keratinocytes (where it is stored). Safe anti-pigmentation agents are expected to inhibit the overactivation of melanin formation while maintaining normal levels of pigment production. Such anti-pigmentation agents suppress melanogenesis without the risk of causing

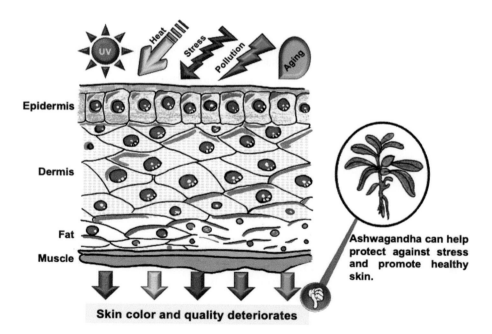

FIGURE 4.7 Diagram showing the bioactivities of Ashwagandha on the skin. Environmental stress and age-related changes in our bodies cause damage to skin cells, resulting in skin darkening. Ashwagandha ingredients protect the skin from stress and improve skin quality. Protection against UV or stress-induced darkening and dryness has been documented.

hypopigmentation in normal skin conditions. Research on the anti-pigmentation activity of Ashwagandha extracts has reported the following results.

- Withaferin A caused marked inhibition of stimulated, but not normal unstimulated, tyrosinase activity.
- Withaferin A blocked both endothelins (EDN1)– and stem cell factor (SCF)–stimulated pigmentation of human epidermal cells in culture. Notably, a decrease in stimulated pigmentation, but not in normal levels, was observed.
- Ashwagandha extracts protected normal human cells in culture from oxidative stress and DNA damage and induced the protein degradation process responsible for the clearance of macromolecular damage (Figure 4.7).

4.24 CANCER

Cancer is a group of complex diseases and is most simply defined as abnormal cell growth. It can start in any part of the body and can even travel from its primary site to multiple secondary sites through a process called metastasis. The development of cancer, called carcinogenesis, is an extremely complex process driven by multiple factors, including genetics, environment, and lifestyle. While most genetic or hereditary cancers occur at an early age, cancers that occur in old age are largely driven by environmental and lifestyle factors.

Despite exponential improvements in cancer diagnosis, treatment, and care in recent decades, there has also been a remarkable increase in cancer incidence. The most common cancers in adults and the elderly are breast, lung, prostate, colorectal, blood, liver, and rectal cancers. While we rarely heard of cancer in the 1980s, today it is predicted that one in three people will develop cancer in their lifetime. By 2020, there are expected to be ~2 million new cancer cases and ~500,000 deaths in the United States alone.

The increased incidence of cancer that we are currently witnessing is often related to the modern industrialized lifestyle with its excessive use of chemicals. The use of pesticides in agriculture, the use of synthetic chemicals in everyday products, the consumption of preservatives and canned foods, and automobile and industrial waste that pollutes air and water are all contributing factors. In addition, modern lifestyles are often characterized by a lack of physical activity and general social and emotional stress. Alternatively, high cancer incidence may be a byproduct of increased human longevity due to improved standards of living, nutrition, and health care. Either reason is likely to contribute to today's high cancer rates. In the past, people in their 50s had high death rates from diabetes and cardiac arrest. However, the prognosis for these conditions has improved remarkably due to better medical and health care, in part due to longer life expectancy. Now these are more common causes of death for people in their 70s, along with cancer.

Research, especially in cell culture models, has helped us understand how cancer develops and how to treat it with drugs. Cytotoxicity of drugs in cultured cells is the first step in anti-cancer drug development. Before describing the characterization of such cytotoxicity of Ashwagandha-derived extracts and constituents, it is worthwhile to understand the basic concepts of these experiments. More details can also be found in specialized research articles and books.

Normal somatic cells in our body have a limited lifespan. After a certain number of divisions, cells enter a state of permanent growth arrest called replicative senescence. Cancer is a disease of proliferation in which normal cells lose this control and divide uncontrollably, resulting in a tumor (Figure 4.8). Research over the past three decades has shown that normal cells have natural mechanisms that prevent them from dividing indefinitely. These mechanisms are controlled by proteins called tumor suppressor proteins.

p53 and pRb are tumor suppressor proteins that act as master controllers of genomic instability and DNA damage repair pathways that are often overactive in cancer cells. In addition to the loss of tumor suppressor protein function, cancer cells often activate another set of proteins called oncogenes that promote cell survival under stress conditions. Based on the established facts that (i) senescence driven by tumor suppressor genes in normal cells inhibits cancer and (ii) tumor suppressor activities are lost in cancer cells, inducing senescence in cancer cells is a valid strategy for their treatment. Cell culture studies have also provided evidence that old cells synthesize and secrete factors that increase their and neighboring cells' risk of becoming cancerous, providing evidence for the link between senescence and carcinogenesis.

Cancer drug development is an expensive, tough, and time-consuming process. Of the 121 prescription anti-cancer drugs (often called chemotherapeutic or chemopreventive agents) in use today, 90 are derived from plants. Between 1981 and 2002, 48 of the 65 drugs approved by the FDA were developed from natural products. Many of the phytochemicals from Ayurvedic herbs contain multiple active components – as opposed to single chemicals in modern medicine – that work together to produce therapeutic benefits with fewer negative side effects.

With three decades of research experience in the basic biology of cellular aging and the discovery of two proteins (mortalin and Collaborator of ARF (CARF/CDKN2AIP) that appeared to be intimately involved in the regulation of cell proliferation, we asked: What next? The challenge was to translate our findings into information that would be useful to society. One conventional way was to initiate drug discovery using these molecules as targets. However, the average estimated cost and time for a cancer clinical trial is about $20 million and 6–7 years. And yet the success rate of any clinical trial is only about 15%. Given these odds, and with the added responsibilities of having students to graduate, basic research funding to secure, and ongoing studies to publish, we were convinced that conventional drug development was not the right path for us.

With a strong desire to bring our research to the public, we decided to do drug development our way. We wanted to look for Naturally Efficient and Welfare (NEW) compounds that could selectively kill cancer cells and be safe or even beneficial for normal cells. So we decided to combine our experience in molecular research with the knowledge of traditional Ayurvedic home medicine. Traditional home medicine elements and modern molecular biology technologies have different niches – the best place to bring them together was in a laboratory equipped with the tools and technologies to create experimentally validated NEW anti-cancer compounds. In light of

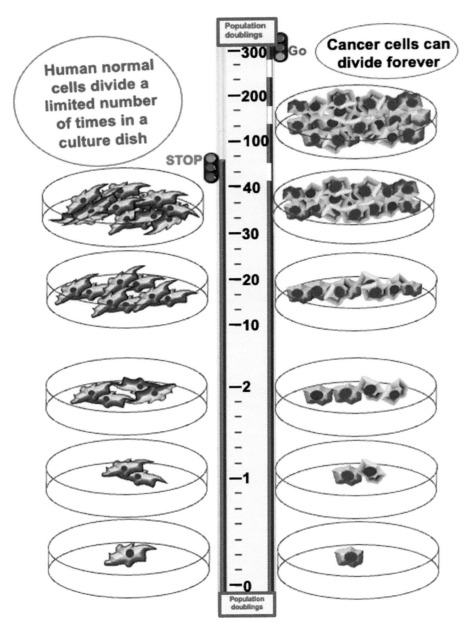

FIGURE 4.8 Graphic representation of normal and cancer cell division. While normal cells stop dividing after a certain fixed number of divisions, cancer cells can divide forever.

the knowledge that stress is intimately linked to aging, age-related pathologies, and cancer, we put considerable thought and effort into searching for anti-stress activities in NEW compounds so that they could be recruited not only to treat cancer but also to improve the overall quality of life. We envisioned that our NEW compounds could reach society without the conventional drug development path and without being limited to patients.

Ashwagandha, the queen of Ayurveda, was our focus. In addition to hearing about Ashwagandha while growing up in India – our parents and grandparents used it for a variety of purposes, including treating colds, inflammation, pain, arthritis, wounds, and fevers – some early clinical studies showed that Ashwagandha could sensitize cancer to radiation therapy. Since we wanted something environmentally and biologically friendly and did not want to be biased in the selection of active ingredients, we decided to prepare both alcoholic and aqueous extracts of Ashwagandha leaves. Alcohol and water extract different compounds from the plant, so these extracts would allow us to separate the active compounds into two broad categories: alcohol-soluble and water-soluble.

Before using the extracts in our cell culture models, we tested the ability of the extracts to stop the growth of tumors in mice. In these experiments, human cancer cells from an aggressive malignant connective tissue tumor called fibrosarcoma are placed under the skin of mice that have a genetically suppressed immune system (called immunodeficient mice). These cells grow into solid tumors in the mice in about 2–3 weeks. We monitored tumor growth daily in control mice fed a normal diet or in test mice fed or injected with Ashwagandha extracts. We thought that these short experiments would help us select the extract with the best anti-cancer activity. To our surprise, we found that both alcohol and water extracts significantly delayed tumor growth. In some experiments, we started feeding/injecting extracts when the tumors were already 1–2 cm in diameter. In these mice treated with alcohol extract, the tumors completely disappeared (Figure 4.9).

To understand the mechanism of Ashwagandha's anti-cancer activity, we used different cultured human cancer cells. The idea was to see if the anti-cancer activity was universal to all cancer cell types or specific to certain types. We grew cells in media containing either alcohol or aqueous extract of Ashwagandha.

Remarkably, the alcohol extract was toxic to all cancer cell types tested. These included breast, lung, brain, and colon cancer cells. Normal cells were not affected, meaning that the alcohol extract was predominantly toxic to cancer cells (Figure 4.10).

We then wanted to know what compounds these extracts contained and which ones selectively killed cancer cells. So we analyzed the chemicals in the extracts using techniques called high-performance liquid chromatography and nuclear magnetic resonance (NMR). These techniques allow scientists to separate and identify the exact compounds in a complex mixture like our extracts. This analysis showed that the extracts contained Wi-A and Wi-N as the main components. Extracts with high levels of Wi-A and Wi-N had higher anti-cancer activity in mouse models. Water extract contained TEG along with low levels of Wi-A.

We again turned to published studies to see if others had studied Wi-A and Wi-N. Indeed, several studies have reported that the active anti-cancer withanolides from Ashwagandha include Wi-A and Wi-N. Other studies show that Wi-A, the most

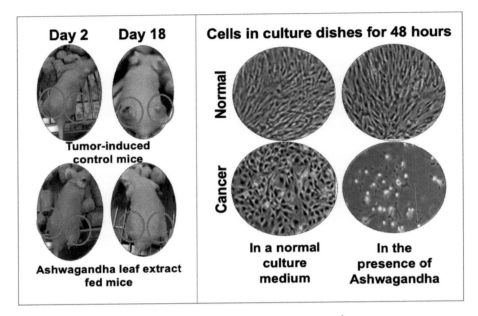

FIGURE 4.9 Anti-cancer activity of Ashwagandha leaf extract. Mice injected with human tumor cells were fed with Ashwagandha extract. While control mice developed large tumors in about 18–20 days, tumor growth was suppressed in Ashwagandha-fed mice (left). Normal and cancer cells were cultured in a dish and treated with Ashwagandha extract. Cancer cells died only in the presence of Ashwagandha extract.

extensively studied of all withanolides, has anti-cancer activity. This was encouraging and motivated us to continue our work. Although several other studies have reported the anti-cancer activity of Wi-A, its mechanism of action remains unknown. We found that, while Wi-N has milder anti-cancer activity, it does not harm normal cells. Interestingly, while Wi-A treatment was toxic to normal cells, the addition of Wi-N along with Wi-A protected the cells.

To identify the cellular targets for anti-cancer activity, we have adopted a unique technology platform used for drug screening called loss-of-function screening. In this screening, we can eliminate proteins from cells either randomly or specifically using molecular scissors called ribozymes or small interfering ribonucleic acid (siRNA), respectively. These compromised cancer cells are then treated with Ashwagandha extracts, and non-responding cells that survive the treatment are analyzed (Figure 4.11).

Using these approaches combined with powerful computational methods, we found that the alcohol extract of Ashwagandha and its components (Wi-A and Wi-N) activate the tumor suppressor protein p53 in cancer cells. Such effects were not observed in normal cells treated with alcohol extract or Wi-N. In contrast, Wi-A, which was cytotoxic to both cancer and normal cells, activated p53 in both cell types. These results were a motivating turning point that seemed to answer our first question of how alcohol extract selectively kills cancer cells. Through multiple experiments

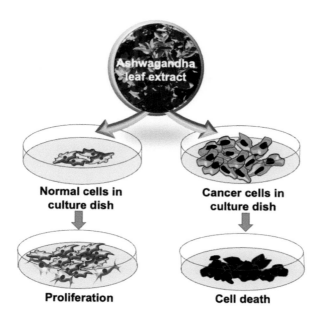

FIGURE 4.10 Graphic representation of the selective killing activity of cancer cells in Ashwagandha leaf extract. Ashwagandha leaf extract was added to the culture medium of normal and cancer cells. Cancer cells but not normal cells died.

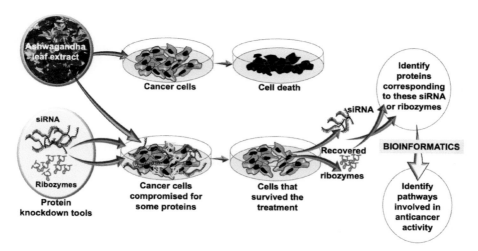

FIGURE 4.11 Schematic diagram showing the experimental design to investigate the molecular mechanism of anti-cancer activity of Ashwagandha extract. Cultured cancer cells are subjected to gene knockdown followed by treatment with Ashwagandha extract. The particular gene knockdown that made the cells resistant to the effect of the extract was considered important for anti-cancer activity and was further studied by advanced bioinformatics and experimental approaches.

analyzing a variety of cancer cell lines and p53, we resolved that alcohol extract and Wi-N are selectively toxic to cancer cells by activating the p53 tumor suppressor.

p53 is a transcription factor, a protein that helps control how a cell reads DNA and translates genetic information into mRNA and proteins. It is considered a guardian of the genome and a master stress regulator because it regulates the activity of many other proteins. It puts cells into dormancy/growth arrest, giving them time to repair genetic damage before they divide. Otherwise, stress-induced genetic damage can amplify and lead to genetic instability that is a hallmark of cancer cells, in which p53 is often mutated and/or functionally inactive. Overall, it is inactivated in more than 80% of cancers. p53 is regulated by several factors that bind to specific parts of the protein. We and others have shown that p53 binds to a stress protein called mortalin, which is enriched in cancer cells. Mortalin resides predominantly in the cytoplasm of cells and holds p53 there, preventing it from entering the nucleus and thereby disabling some of its normal transcriptional activation and tumor suppressor functions. Treating cells with the alcohol extract of Ashwagandha interrupts the mortalin–p53 interaction and allows p53 to return to its nucleus and resume its tumor suppressor action preventing the growth of cancer cells and causing their death. Interestingly, treating cancer cells with alcohol extract also affects the protein mortalin, which is used as a marker to identify normal or cancer cells. The location of mortalin is altered in cancer cells; it is seen as a widely distributed protein in the cytoplasm of normal cells, but, in cancer cells, it is localized predominantly in the perinuclear region. Treating cancer cells with Ashwagandha extract returns mortalin to the pattern seen in normal cells. This shift was again a pleasant and encouraging surprise, as it also related to our other ongoing research projects. A similar change in the subcellular distribution of mortalin was found when cancer cells were induced to undergo senescence-like growth arrest in response to treatment with a rhodacyanine dye (MKT-077 and its derivatives), bromodeoxyuridine (BrdU), single chromosomes encoding tumor suppressor proteins, caffeic acid phenethyl ester and artepillin C (active components of honey bee propolis), and cucurbitacin B (an active component of bitter cucumber and Chinese ginseng). All of these inhibit mortalin–p53 complexes, causing p53 to move to the nucleus and turn p53 on, causing cells to stop growing. In some cases, high doses of reagents cause cell death.

Next, we dug deeper to understand the mechanism of action of Wi-A and Wi-N, using molecular tools and bioinformatics (computational studies) to see if these molecules dock to the p53–mortalin complex. Molecular docking is a powerful tool in structural molecular biology and computer-aided drug design. Simply put, we can analyze the structure of proteins and compounds and determine how they best fit together. By docking Wi-A and Wi-N to the mortalin and p53 proteins, we discovered that these small molecules were able to interfere with the mortalin–p53 protein interaction. This interference was expected to push p53 back into the nucleus, activating its DNA transcription and growth arrest functions. In our experiments, cancer cells treated with Wi-A and Wi-N did indeed show p53 in the nucleus and growth arrest/cell death. At the molecular level, these effects were seen to be mediated by an increase in proteins that cause growth arrest (p21WAF1) and apoptosis (Bax). Of note, since the mortalin–p53 interaction occurs only in cancer cells (normal cells lack this interaction), these data explain the selective toxicity to cancer cells.

The results show that the alcohol extract of Ashwagandha has anti-cancer activity by blocking mortalin–p53 interactions, activating normal p53 function as evidenced by an increase in p21WAF1 protein, and inducing senescence-like growth arrest in cancer cells (Figure 4.12).

Since most cancer cells (~80%) have mutations in p53, our next intriguing question was how anti-cancer activity applies in such a scenario that requires normal p53 function. We studied cancer cells with mutant p53 protein. Treating these cells with an alcoholic extract of Ashwagandha resulted in decreased levels of mutant p53 protein. This was an exciting observation because mutant p53 is stable and accumulates in cancer cells, and a lot of research has looked for drugs that can break down mutant p53 – we were excited to find that Ashwagandha leaf extract is capable of such a function. Scientists searching for new anti-cancer drugs have also been looking for compounds that make mutant p53 act more like normal p53 so that it causes growth arrest and death of cancer cells. Based on this concept, and with our fingers crossed, we performed p53-specific experiments in cells treated with alcohol extract. The results were positive – mutant p53 acquired normal p53 activity in alcohol extract-treated cancer cells, stopping cell growth and even causing cell death.

The next obvious question was whether the mutant-to-normal reversal would work for all types of p53 mutants. Several p53 mutations induce localized or more widespread changes in protein structure that affect how the protein binds to DNA. Structural differences between normal and mutant p53 provide an opportunity to selectively target cancer cells with mutant p53. Although restoring normal p53 activity in mutants with small molecules can reverse the structural changes, not all mutants behave similarly. Therefore, we next used docking tools and bioinformatics to investigate the structural changes between normal and mutant p53 proteins.

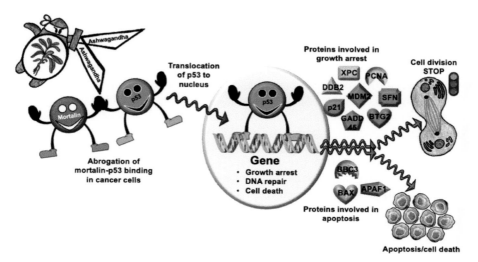

FIGURE 4.12 Schematic diagram showing how Ashwagandha extract blocks the mortalin–p53 interaction in cancer cells, thereby allowing p53 to enter the nucleus where it functions to activate various proteins causing either growth arrest (top) or apoptosis (bottom).

We investigated the therapeutic potential of Wi-A and Wi-N to restore several specific p53 mutants (p53V143A, p53R249S, p53R273H, and p53Y220C) to normal p53. Extensive molecular docking analyses showed that the p53V143A mutation does not have significant structural changes and does not allow binding by witha-nolides. The p53R249S mutation disrupts binding to destabilize the DNA binding site. However, withanolides did not show selective binding to this mutant or other similar variants. The p53Y220C mutation created a cavity near the mutation site, resulting in a dysfunctional protein. The mutant, but not the normal, structure could accommodate withanolides, suggesting the selectivity of the compounds to target the p53Y220C mutant. Using human cell lines containing specific p53 mutant pro-teins, we performed experiments and demonstrated that Wi-A, Wi-N, and extract rich in these withanolides restored normal p53 function in p53Y220C mutant cells and induced growth arrest and apoptosis by activating p21WAF-1 function. These results suggest that withanolides may be potent anti-cancer agents for the treatment of cancers harboring a specific p53Y220C mutation.

At this point, we were happy to have recruited our unique molecular technologies to gain insight into how the alcohol extract of Ashwagandha selectively kills cancer cells. Some of the other leads that emerged from this functional screening included GADD45 and TPX2. GADD45 is a protein involved in DNA damage response and repair; it is activated in response to DNA damage and blocks cell proliferation. In fact, through experiments, we found that the cells treated with the alcoholic extract of Ashwagandha possess a higher amount of GADD45 and thereby they stop dividing. TPX2 is a protein associated with a structural protein, tubulin, which is essential for the process of cell division (driven by several factors, regulated in a controlled and coordinated way). Cells go through a preparatory phase (synthesis phase – S and gap phases – G1 and G2) before entering the actual cell division phase, which is called mitosis. During mitosis, the genetic material (chromosomes) divides into two sets that eventually give rise to two "daughter" cells. TPX2 forms a protein complex with Aurora A to distribute the genetic material to the two daughter cells. Both TPX2 and Aurora A proteins and their complex are enriched in cancer cells, where they play a critical role in rapid cell proliferation. Using computational and experimental assays, we discovered that Wi-A can bind to and dissociate the TPX2-Aurora A complex, resulting in the disruption of cell division in cancer cells (Figure 4.13).

Another category of the functional mechanism of anti-cancer activity of Ashwagandha seemed to be oxidative stress on cancer cells. This led us to inves-tigate whether cellular stress signaling was activated in cells treated with alcohol extract. The amount of ROS in cells is a sign of oxidative stress and can be measured in living cells using fluorescent dyes (Figure 4.14). Increased levels of ROS lead to (i) mitochondrial stress leading to changes in membrane potential and (ii) DNA damage stress leading to activation of the DNA damage and repair machinery.

We examined both types of stress in alcohol extract-treated cells. To exam-ine mitochondrial stress, we examined the structure of untreated and alcohol extract-treated cells using a high-resolution microscope. Cancer cells have a standard mitochondrial structure characterized by a membrane that is neatly folded and orga-nized in a maze-like pattern (Figure 4.15). Cells treated with Ashwagandha alcohol extract instead had swollen mitochondria with an altered structure of shorter and

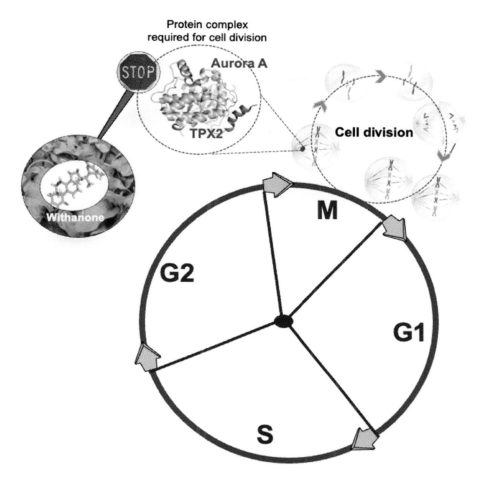

FIGURE 4.13 Schematic diagram showing how Ashwagandha extract and withanone inhibit the Aurora A–TPX2 protein complex, thereby blocking cancer cell division.

fewer membrane folds (called cristae). In addition, DNA damage markers γH2AX and p53BP1, which increase in response to DNA damage stress, were elevated in alcohol extract-treated cells.

DNA damage is closely linked to the aging process. Telomere shortening causes DNA damage that eventually puts cells in a state of permanent growth arrest. Telomeres are specialized protein caps at the ends of our chromosomes. These structures have several important biological functions, including preventing chromosome ends from sticking together and keeping genetic material stable. Telomeres play a key role in regulating gene expression, senescence of normal cells, and immortality of cancer cells. In normal cells, telomeres gradually shorten each time the cell divides. In contrast, cancer cells activate an enzyme called telomerase, which can lengthen telomeres. Many cancers express telomerase, so compounds that inhibit telomerase are predicted to work as cancer therapies. However, some cancer cells (~10%–15%

**Cancer cells in culture stained for
Reactive Oxygen Species (ROS)**

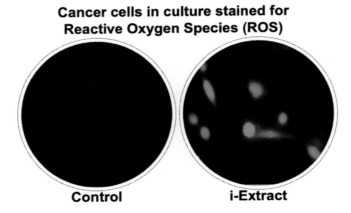

Control   **i-Extract**

FIGURE 4.14 Cancer cells cultured in a medium containing Ashwagandha extract show high levels of reactive oxygen species (ROS), seen as a green color, indicating their oxidatively stressed state.

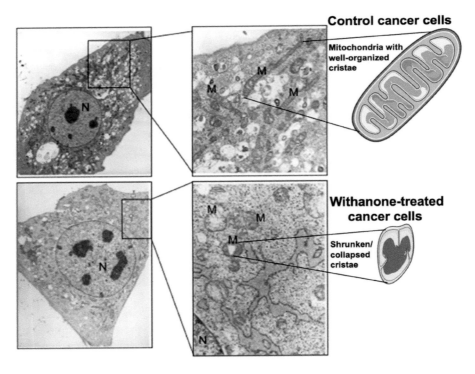

FIGURE 4.15 Cancer cells cultured in a medium containing Ashwagandha extract show mitochondrial damage. While the control cancer cells showed long cylindrical, well-organized cristae, the treated cells showed shrunken, rounded mitochondria that stained green, indicating their oxidatively stressed state (Widodo et al., 2010).

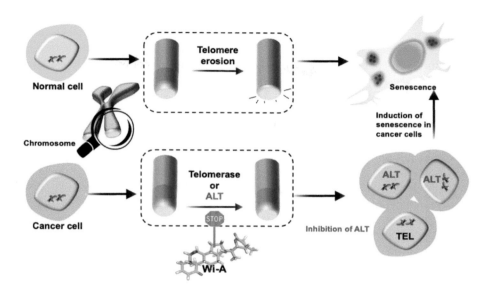

FIGURE 4.16 Diagram of telomere shortening in normal cells. Cancer cells maintain their telomeres either by activating the enzyme telomerase or by an alternative mechanism called ALT. The Ashwagandha constituent withaferin A (Wi-A) blocks ALT.

of cancers, especially sarcomas and astrocytomas) maintain their telomeres without telomerase. These cells instead use a mechanism called alternative lengthening of telomeres, often abbreviated as ALT. Cancers with activated ALT are unlikely to respond to telomerase inhibitors. Cancers can also have cells with telomerase turned on as well as cells with ALT. In these cancers, inhibiting telomerase alone may not be an effective treatment. This creates a need for dual inhibitors of telomerase and ALT.

Using similar cultured cancer cell lines expressing either telomerase or ALT, we found that Wi-A has stronger cytotoxic effects on ALT cells than on telomerase-expressing cells. Wi-A blocks proteins involved in ALT, suggesting that Wi-A is a candidate inhibitor for ALT cancers (Figure 4.16).

After discovering the anti-cancer activity of the alcohol extract of Ashwagandha leaf and its mechanism of action, we began to think about its application. Clearly, the alcohol extract seemed a better choice than Wi-A alone because of its toxicity to normal cells, and Wi-N was not as potent. One hurdle that still needed to be worked out was the alcohol extraction, as this is not something that can be easily done in the kitchen. So we thought it was obvious to see if we could isolate the compounds more easily using an inexpensive, convenient, and safe alternative – water.

After trying several methods, we prepared water extracts to test anti-cancer potential in cultured human cells and mouse tumor models. Immunodeficient mice fed 500 mg/kg body weight of Ashwagandha water extract every other day for 60 days showed no toxicity in terms of changes in body weight and physical activity. After implanting human fibrosarcoma cells under the skin, we fed the mice 250 mg/kg bw of water extract every other day and monitored tumor growth. In about 20 days,

21 of 24 control mice developed large tumors, while one had a small tumor and two had no tumors. On the contrary, mice fed Ashwagandha water extract showed strong tumor suppression. In this group of 24 mice, 12 had no tumors, 3 had small clusters of tumor cells (called tumor buds), 5 had small tumors, and only 4 developed large tumors. In the lung metastasis model, water extract–fed mice also had fewer cancer metastases. There were less than 5 metastatic tumors in water extract–fed mice, whereas control mice had more than 50 metastatic tumors. These results suggest that the water extract has significant anti-cancer activity in both cultured cells and mouse models. However, the analysis of the chemicals in Ashwagandha water extract showed that it contains low levels of Wi-A and Wi-N – opening a new chapter for us.

With great curiosity, we conducted experiments to separate and identify individual components of the extract using a technique called NMR. Unexpectedly, we identified a small compound called TEG as a potent component that suppressed tumor growth in mice. TEG is well established as a low-toxicity, mild disinfectant for a variety of airborne, solution-, and surface-bound microbes, including bacteria and viruses. An old study in dogs with inoperable malignant and metastatic tonsillar epithelioma and reticular cell sarcoma reported that tumors regressed in response to TEG treatment without toxicity (Figure 4.17).

Analysis of the anti-cancer activity of TEG revealed that it activates the p53 and pRb tumor suppressor pathways. However, in contrast to the selective activation of p53 in response to the alcohol extract of Ashwagandha, the water extract activated p53 in both cancer and normal cells. Instead, the pRb tumor suppressor was activated only in cancer cells. The pRb protein works closely with the E2F family of

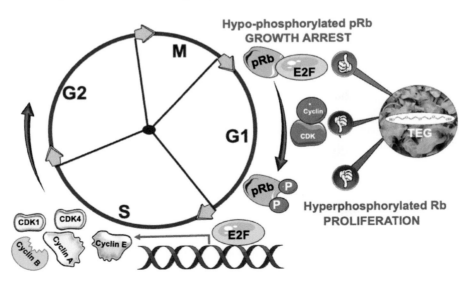

FIGURE 4.17 Schematic showing the effect of TEG on cancer cell proliferation through the activation of the pRB tumor suppressor protein. While in cancer cells pRB is phosphorylated and does not block E2F from its cell cycle–promoting function, Ashwagandha-treated cancer cells show inhibition of pRB phosphorylation. In its hypophosphorylated state, pRB binds to E2F and blocks its cell cycle–promoting function.

transcription factors to promote cell division. By binding to E2F proteins, pRb inhibits several proteins required for cell division. Cell cycle inhibitors modify pRb with a phosphate group, called phosphorylation, which changes pRb's activity by separating it from E2F. E2F then becomes active and stimulates cells to divide. Cells treated with alcohol extract have more dephosphorylated pRb, which actively interacts with E2F and inhibits its function. Several other proteins in this pathway are altered in treated cells, halting cell growth.

Our results not only demonstrated the molecular basis of the anti-cancer activity in the leaves of Ashwagandha but also provided compelling evidence that the whole herb provides better activity than its extracts or individual components. We learned from our experiments that (i) the bioactive components in alcohol and water extracts of Ashwagandha are different, and (ii) although both types of extracts possess anti-cancer activity, their mechanism of action and target proteins are different. Thus, to obtain the full spectrum of activities and ensure multi-target action, it is reasonable to consume leaf powder rather than separate extracted compounds for cancer management (Figure 4.18).

For this reason, we thought that Ashwagandha leaf powder might offer a full spectrum of activity and therefore provide a more effective cancer treatment. Since cells cannot be fed with leaf powder, we went back to our mouse models to test the anti-cancer activity of Ashwagandha leaf powder on human fibrosarcoma cells injected under the skin of immunosuppressed mice. Feeding the mice Ashwagandha leaf powder (500 mg/kg body weight) showed no toxicity or negative side effects, but strongly suppressed tumor growth. Since we did not know how much of the active anti-cancer ingredients could be accessed by the body, we tried to improve their availability by using cyclodextrins. Cyclodextrins, widely used in the pharmaceutical industry, are circular sugars that can encapsulate small molecules and improve their

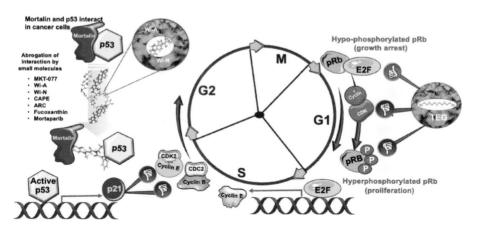

FIGURE 4.18 Schematic diagram showing the effect of TEG on cancer cell proliferation through the activation of the pRB tumor suppressor protein. While in cancer cells pRB is phosphorylated and does not block E2F from its cell cycle–promoting function, Ashwagandha-treated cancer cells show inhibition of pRB phosphorylation. In its hypophosphorylated state, pRB binds to E2F and blocks its cell cycle–promoting function.

stability and bioavailability. Indeed, our experiments combining Ashwagandha leaf powder with cyclodextrin showed greater tumor suppression in immunosuppressed mice (Figure 4.19). These experimental results indicate that Ashwagandha leaf powder, together with cyclodextrin, provides better anti-cancer benefits.

Still curious to know what other treasures the herb held, we analyzed Ashwagandha extracts some more. Interestingly, the extract contained a close relative of Wi-A called 2,3-dihydro-3β-methoxy Wi-A (3βmWi-A). Since Wi-A is the most potent anti-cancer component in Ashwagandha leaves, we eagerly investigated the activity of 3βmWi-A in our cultured cells. To our surprise, 3βmWi-A was not toxic to normal human cells. In biochemical and imaging analyses, while Wi-A causes oxidative stress in normal cells, 3βmWi-A is well tolerated even at tenfold higher concentrations. We were surprised to find that it promotes survival and protects normal cells exposed to oxidative, UV, and chemical stress (Figure 4.20).

In this way, another mystery of nature came to light – both toxic ingredients and their antidotes are present together in the plant. Extensive analysis revealed that (i) 3βmWi-A, rather than Wi-A, is safe and can alleviate stress; (ii) 3βmWi-A, when administered after stressors including Wi-A, protects normal cells from toxicity; and (iii) 3βmWi-A is an important compound that may protect normal cells from

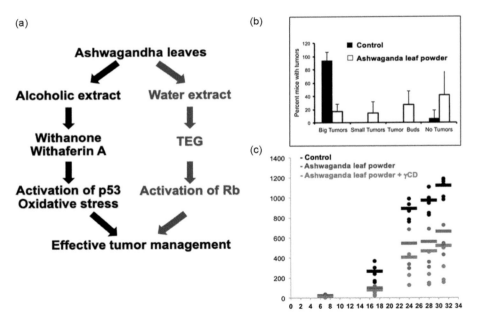

FIGURE 4.19 Schematics show that Ashwagandha leaves contain a variety of anti-cancer compounds that act through different mechanisms. Withanone and withaferin A cause activation of the p53 tumor suppressor protein, and TEG causes activation of the pRB tumor suppressor protein. Together, they provide enhanced anti-cancer activity (A). Feeding tumor-bearing mice with Ashwagandha leaf powder caused effective suppression of tumors (B) and feeding γCD along with Ashwagandha leaf powder was more effective (C) (Wadhwa et al., 2017).

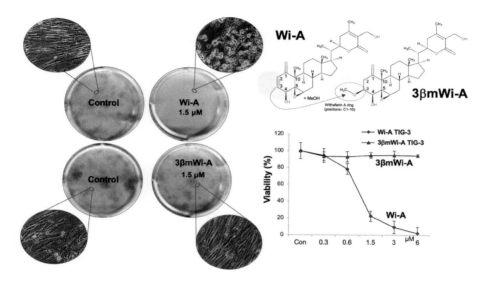

FIGURE 4.20 Cell culture dishes in which cancer cells were cultured in either control or Wi-A/ 3βmWi-A supplemented medium. As can be seen in the enlarged images, Wi-A killed cancer cells, while 3βmWi-A had no effect (left). The two compounds have a small difference in structure (top right) but a large difference in their ability to kill cancer cells (bottom right) (Chaudhary et al., 2017).

the toxicity of targeted therapeutics in clinical practice. Overall, we discovered that 3βmWi-A is an anti-stress and pro-survival factor that co-exists with the anti-cancer compounds in Ashwagandha leaves (Figure 4.21).

- Over the past decade, many additional studies have provided experimental evidence and molecular insights into the anti-cancer bioactive compounds in Ashwagandha leaves. While further studies are needed to determine their efficacy in clinical models of cancer and to identify exactly how they work in the human body, some results relevant to anti-cancer activity are summarized below.
- Several studies in cell and mouse models have reported growth inhibitory effects of Wi-A on B-cell lymphoma, leukemia, and myelodysplastic syndrome.
- Purified Wi-A has anti-inflammatory and immunostimulatory properties. Normal mice respond to Wi-A-rich extracts by increasing cytokine production, suggesting immune-enhancing effects.
- Human immune cells produce inducible nitric oxide synthase (iNOS) when stimulated by pro-inflammatory signals. iNOS protects against many pathogens, including bacteria, fungi, viruses, and parasites. Wi-A stimulates iNOS production by macrophages, which may account for some of its immunostimulatory properties.
- Ashwagandha extract enhances both cell-mediated and humoral immunity by increasing cytokine expression. Oral administration of crude root

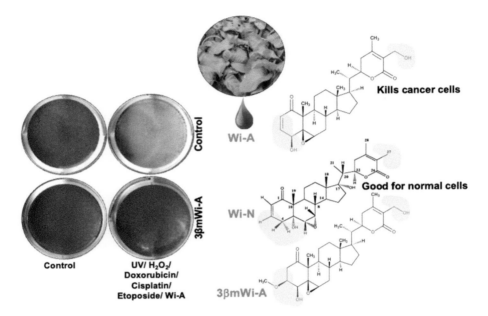

FIGURE 4.21 Cell culture dishes in which normal/stressed cells were cultured in either control or 3βmWi-A-supplemented medium. As seen, the stressed control cells died while the cells cultured with 3βmWi-A survived. These experiments and the others described above showed that Wi-A has anti-cancer activity, and Wi-N and 3βmWi-A are good for normal cells.

extracts or purified Wi-A protected hamsters against infection with *Brugia malayi* or *Leishmania donovani* parasites. Animals fed Wi-A extract had increased levels of iNOS, IFN-γ, IL-12, and TNF-α.

- NF-κB is a multifunctional transcription factor that regulates inflammation, cytokine production, stress response, apoptosis, and tumorigenesis. Ashwagandha extract has been shown to inhibit NF-κB function by blocking its translocation to the nucleus and preventing direct binding to DNA. In addition, Wi-A inactivated inflammatory signaling by preventing the activation of NF-κB nuclear translocation of NF-κB. Reduction of NF-κB activity in Wi-A-treated B lymphoma cells was reported. Wi-A also stops the growth of cancer cells by activating oxidative stress and DNA damage response signaling.

- Wi-A causes the collapse of the protein vimentin, which regulates cell shape and migration and is critical for cancer metastasis. It also blocks the snail and E-cadherin proteins, which send signals that allow cells to become more invasive.

- In human cervical cancer cells, Wi-A silences human papillomavirus proteins that promote cancer and restore p53 function, stopping cell growth or causing cell death.

- Wi-A sensitizes human cancer cells to radiation therapy and works in combination with other anti-cancer drugs, including sorafenib, oxaliplatin, and cisplatin.

- Non-Hodgkin's lymphoma, which originates from a type of immune cell called a B-cell, accounts for more than 4% of all cancers in the United States. Diffuse large B-cell lymphoma is one of the most common and aggressive forms of non-Hodgkin's lymphoma, accounting for 30% of newly diagnosed cases of B-cell lymphoma. Current therapy for diffuse large B-cell lymphoma includes the R-CHOP regimen (rituximab, cyclophosphamide, doxorubicin, vincristine, and prednisone), which often leads to the development of treatment resistance with ~40% patient mortality. Wi-A is effective against diffuse large B-cell lymphoma in mouse models.
- Non-Hodgkin's lymphomas can be classified into aggressive and fast-growing types (diffuse large B-cell lymphoma, mantle cell lymphoma, and Burkitt's lymphoma) or slow-growing types (chronic lymphocytic leukemia and follicular lymphoma). Chronic lymphocytic leukemia is the most common adult leukemia in the Western world. Unlike many diffuse large B-cell lymphomas, which are characterized by uncontrolled growth, the leukemic cells are abnormal lymphocytes that have defects in cell death mechanisms, causing the cells to accumulate. In mouse models of chronic lymphocytic leukemia, Wi-A inhibited cell growth and triggered cell death mechanisms.
- Wi-A blocks proliferation, angiogenesis, and metastasis and induces apoptosis and autophagy in a variety of cell culture models (Figure 4.22).

4.25 CANCER METASTASIS

Metastasis is a complex process regulated by multiple interactions of genetic and environmental factors. In metastasis, cancer cells travel through the bloodstream to spread from a tumor to other sites in the body. Metastasis is regulated by the characteristics of tumor cells as well as the environment surrounding a tumor. It poses major hurdles to cancer therapy. The choice of cancer treatment (surgery, chemotherapy, radiation therapy, hormone therapy, laser immunotherapy, or a combination of these) depends on the type of primary cancer, its size, and the location of metastases.

The most direct cancer treatment is surgical removal of the tumor. Other treatments include reducing tumor growth with synthetic or herbal drugs that are taken orally, injected, or applied to the tumor as a paste. These either act directly on the cancer or promote deeper healing by supporting the immune system. In most cases, chemotherapy is used, which includes multiple drugs to kill cancer cells and boost the immune system. However, treatment is complicated by metastasis. It is the cause of tumor recurrence in 90% of cancers, leading to treatment failure and a high risk of death. Current options for curing metastatic cancers are very limited. There is a great need to better understand metastasis, to discover how cells migrate and contact each other, and to formulate new strategies for safe and effective cancer treatment.

The process of metastasis requires:

i. Epithelial-to-mesenchymal transition is a process by which one cell type changes into another cell type that can migrate and is more invasive. In this process, epithelial cells undergo drastic molecular and structural changes

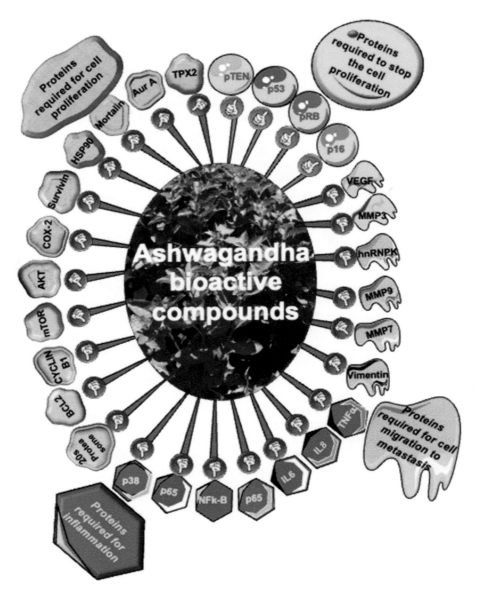

FIGURE 4.22 A portrait of the protein targets of Ashwagandha constituents – withanone, withaferin A, and TEG. The proteins involved in cancer cell proliferation migration and inflammation are largely affected. Of note, tumor suppressor proteins that stop cell proliferation are upregulated and oncogenic proteins that promote proliferation are downregulated. Together, these bring cancer cell division to a halt. Proteins required for migration, invasion, and metastasis as well as inflammation are decreased.

to become mesenchymal cells. Epithelial cells are tightly connected to each other, but mesenchymal cells only interact with each other at certain points. Ashwagandha and Wi-A inhibit epithelial-to-mesenchymal transition.

ii. Tumor cells acquire migratory properties so that they can move away from the primary tumor site. Ashwagandha and Wi-A inhibit the migration of cancer cells.

iii. Metastatic cells can break down surrounding connective tissue and enter the bloodstream, where they can travel to distant sites in the body and form new tumors. Ashwagandha and Wi-A block the invasion and angiogenic properties of cancer cells.

iv. Enzymes called matrix metalloproteinases regulate the extracellular matrix that surrounds cells and play an important role in tumor metastasis and angiogenesis. These enzymes, in turn, are regulated by cytokines and growth factors through interconnected signaling pathways. Ashwagandha and Wi-A inhibit the activities of these proteins.

As discussed, a large body of experimental evidence led us to believe that Wi-A and Wi-N have anti-cancer activity. We wanted to further test whether these compounds could prevent cancer cells from migrating from a primary tumor to metastatic sites. To metastasize, cancer cells must be able to migrate, invade surrounding tissue, and form new blood vessels. Laboratory tests can measure these characteristics. Cell migration is measured using a "wound scratch" assay. In this experiment, cells are grown in a single layer in the laboratory. A "wound" is created by scratching the layer of cells. We then use a microscope to see if cells move into the scratched area and measure how many cells do so. The ability of cells to invade other tissues is measured in an invasion assay. In this assay, we measure whether cultured cells can pass through special membranes. The ability of cancer cells to form new blood vessels, a process called angiogenesis, is measured in "tube formation" assays. In these experiments, cells are grown in a special matrix and we measure their ability to form blood vessel-like tubes. Using all of these assays in our laboratory, we found that Ashwagandha's bioactive compounds exhibited remarkable anti-migration, anti-invasion, and anti-angiogenic activities. Further testing in mouse models also showed that mice injected with cancer cells and then treated with Ashwagandha extracts had less lung metastasis than untreated mice.

We used these assays to test a combination of Wi-N and Wi-A for anti-migration, anti-invasion, and anti-angiogenic activities. Cultured cells treated with metastasis-inducing compounds [such as vascular endothelial growth factor (VEGF) treatment] were exposed to either standard anti-metastasis drugs or Wi-N/Wi-A. Experiments using bioinformatics and biochemical approaches showed that the combination of Wi-N and Wi-A reduced the levels of migration-promoting proteins (hnRNP-K, VEGF, and metalloproteases) and had effects similar to the anti-metastasis drugs used in the clinic (Figure 4.23).

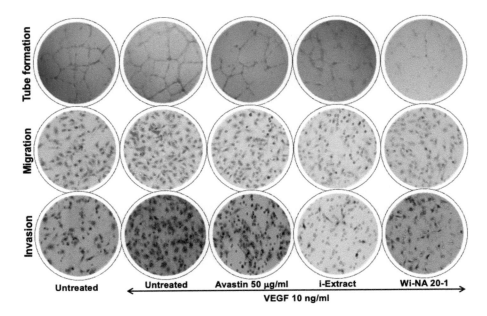

FIGURE 4.23 Cell culture dishes showing cancer cell characteristics (tube formation, migration, and invasion). VEGF caused an increase in all these characteristics, and Ashwagandha caused inhibition. Of note, the inhibition caused by Ashwagandha extract (i-Extract) and the combination of withanone and withaferin A was comparable/even stronger than a clinically used drug Avastin (Gao et al., 2014).

4.26 BRAIN MALIGNANCIES

Several research studies have reported that Ashwagandha has cytotoxic and tumor-sensitizing properties for brain cancer. Based on this, we tested the response of brain-derived cultured cells to alcohol extracts of Ashwagandha, Wi-N, Wi-A, and TEG. In these experiments, cells from two types of brain cancer, glioblastoma and neuroblastoma, showed differentiation and senescence-like growth arrest. These results suggested that we had added a function to the cancer cells to stop them from dividing. This is called differentiation therapy, and it is less toxic to tissues that cannot be removed or treated with radiation therapy.

In our experiments, cells treated with Ashwagandha bioactive compounds had increased expression of proteins involved in the differentiation of glial and neural cells. Treatment with an aqueous extract of Ashwagandha leaves also induced cell differentiation and protected brain-derived cells from damage caused by overexcitation with the neurotransmitter glutamate. Ashwagandha treatment also caused a decrease in proteins normally found in metastatic glioma cells. These included VEGF, PSA-NCAM, HSP70, and cyclin D1 protein. Water extract caused remarkable differentiation in neuroblastoma and glioblastoma. By pre-treating differentiated cells with water extract, we found that the cells were protected from oxidative and glutamate stress. This finding suggests the therapeutic potential of Ashwagandha water extract against neurodegeneration caused by glutamate-induced overexcitation.

Treatment of brain disorders depends in part on the ability of compounds to cross a special barrier called the blood–brain barrier. This tissue separates the blood from the cerebrospinal fluid in the brain. A mouse study showed the presence of withanamides in the blood and brain of mice treated with Ashwagandha extract, indicating that bioactive compounds of Ashwagandha can cross this barrier and enter the brain. Feeding water extract of Ashwagandha leaves also reduced the volume of glioma tumors in a rat model. In fact, aqueous extract of Ashwagandha leaves inhibits the proliferation of human neuroblastoma cells in culture by arresting the cell cycle and inducing cell death. Cells treated with alcoholic extract of Ashwagandha showed activation of several proteins and molecular pathways that promote apoptosis and suppress tumor-promoting proteins. Water extract also caused human neuroblastoma cells to differentiate, inducing structural changes (increased expression of neurofilament 200 and NCAM expression) and anti-metastatic signaling levels (downregulation of MMP3 and MMP9).

Gliomas are the most common type of primary brain tumor in adults. They are aggressive, diverse, and often unresponsive to treatment, resulting in high mortality rates. Based on the anti-proliferative and differentiation-inducing properties of Ashwagandha extracts on cultured neurons, researchers tested the therapeutic potential of Ashwagandha aqueous extract for glioblastoma using a model of glioma cells implanted in the rat brain. After 21 days, control rats had movement problems, appearing slow and dull and turning in only one direction. However, rats fed water extract were healthy, active, and responsive. While control rats developed large tumors, water extract–fed rats had no such visible tumors. When the brains of the rats were examined under a microscope, the tumors in the control rats had metastasized and spread throughout the brain. However, water extract–fed rats had only small, localized tumors. Molecular analysis of these tumors showed a decrease in proteins involved in metastasis and an increase in proteins involved in differentiation. These data suggest that Ashwagandha aqueous extract may be effective for differentiation therapy of metastatic brain tumors.

4.27 FOLIC ACID RECEPTOR–MEDIATED TARGETING ENHANCES THE CYTOTOXICITY, EFFICACY, AND SELECTIVITY OF *WITHANIA SOMNIFERA* LEAF EXTRACT

Given the growing body of experimental data supporting (i) the anti-cancer potential of Ashwagandha leaf extracts, (ii) the identification of bioactive constituents, and (iii) their mechanisms of action, researchers sought to increase this activity by either cultivating plants or developing extraction techniques with enriched levels of anti-cancer compounds. At the same time, nanotechnologies have been created to (i) safeguard the chemicals from deterioration; (ii) improve their bioavailability; and (iii) broaden their cancer cell selectivity. In this regard, over the course of more than 10 years of research, we have created not just distinctive Ashwagandha cultivars with high levels of active withanolides but also water-based extraction techniques with improved anti-cancer potential.

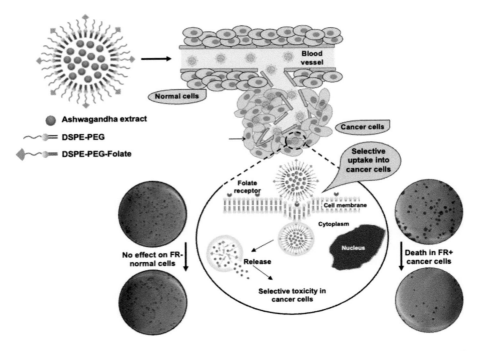

FIGURE 4.24 Schematic presentation of a nano complex formed through self-assembly of amphiphilic block copolymers (DSPE-PEG) with folate ligands that are selectively taken up by cancer cells expressing the folic acid receptor, leading to anti-cancer activity. Normal or cancer cells that lack folic acid receptor expression remain unaffected (Yu et al., 2019).

The use of nanocarriers that can successfully encapsulate tiny molecules based on their various physicochemical properties, including size, charge, hydrophilicity, and hydrophobicity, is employed to further increase the therapeutic potential of chosen extracts. For instance, covering pharmaceuticals with polyethylene glycol (PEG) improves their therapeutic effects. Certain nanocarriers, such as fatty acids, glycols, and pyrrolidones, increase the permeability of active substances through the skin. Additionally, bioactive chemicals can be delivered specifically by being combined with ligands for particular cell surface receptors that are only expressed on target tumor cells. Folic acid therapy that targets the glycosylphosphatidylinositol-anchored glycoprotein folate receptor alpha (FRα), which is overexpressed in 90% of epithelial malignancies, is one example. Through receptor-mediated intracellular transit of its associated bioactive components, folic acid binds to FRα-mediated endocytosis. The low amount of FRα expression in normal cells and tissues allows anti-cancer drugs to target only cancer cells, reducing pan-toxicity and undesirable side effects. Our Ashwagandha leaf extract and folic acid–based folate receptor–targeting nanocomplex (FRi-Ex) exhibit threefold greater cellular absorption in cell-based assays and stronger tumor growth inhibition in mouse models, which was corroborated by biochemical analyses (Figure 4.24).

5 Anti-cancer Ingredients and Their Mechanisms of Action

More than a decade passed as we explored Ashwagandha's bioactive compounds, bioactivities, and mechanism of action. Several other laboratories also reported new findings, identifying active compounds and their target proteins. Among various active ingredients, alkaloids (such as isopelletierine, anaferine, cuscohygrine, anahygrine), steroidal lactones (withanolides, withaferins), and saponins have been repeatedly recognized as important anti-cancer agents that block proteins that regulate cancer cell proliferation and migration. Of these, withaferin A has emerged as a lead candidate.

- Withaferin A causes degradation of the vimentin protein by binding directly to vimentin. Withaferin A-treated cells have disrupted microtubules and microfilaments and increased actin stress fibers, suggesting a stressed state that halts cell growth and causes cell death.
- Withaferin A targets the catalytic subunit of enzymes that break down proteins, called proteasomes, slowing protein degradation to increase pro-apoptotic proteins that kill cancer cells.
- Withaferin A is predicted to block survivin, a protein that regulates cancer cell division, migration, angiogenesis, and chemotherapy resistance. Survivin prevents apoptosis and turns on cell survival and migration signals. Enriched in cancer cells, survivin is associated with advanced tumor stages and metastasis.
- Withaferin A blocks mortalin–p53 interactions that are unique to cancer cells and lead to inactivation of p53 functions. Mortalin is expressed in cancer cells and plays an important role in human carcinogenesis due to its pro-proliferative, anti-apoptotic, and pro-migration activities. Mortalin turns on the telomerase enzyme and the heterogeneous nuclear ribonucleoprotein K (hnRNP-K) protein, contributing to the malignancy of cancer cells. Downregulation of mortalin by withaferin A activates p53, leading to growth arrest or cell death.
- Withaferin A blocks the activity of heat shock protein 90 (HSP90), an abundant protein in cancer cells that helps to assemble or disassemble other proteins. HSP90 inhibitors prevent cancer cell proliferation.
- Withaferin A inhibits metastasis by targeting hnRNP-K and vascular endothelial growth factor proteins, which are essential for cell migration. A combination of withanone and withaferin A at a ratio of 20:1 (WiNA

DOI: 10.1201/9781032705743-5

20–1) was shown to be selectively toxic to cancer cells. Withanone–withaferin A treatment also significantly reduced migration, invasion, and metastasis of cultured fibrosarcoma cells. In tube formation assays, withanone–withaferin A combination blocked tube formation similarly to the antiangiogenic drug Avastin (50 µg/ml). Anti-metastatic activity was also demonstrated in mouse models. Injecting either withanone (1 mg/kg), withaferin A (0.5 mg/kg) or their combination into subcutaneous xenograft and lung metastasis mouse models using human fibrosarcoma (HT1080) also showed anti-cancer and anti-metastasis activity. These mice have lower activity of hnRNP-K protein in treated tumors compared to untreated control tumors. While there were no significant differences in body weight of control, withaferin A, withanone, and WiNA-injected mice. Mice injected with withanone–withaferin A show strong suppression of subcutaneous fibrosarcoma tumors. In a lung metastasis model, large lung tumors were detected only in control mice, suggesting that withanone–withaferin A has potent anti-cancer and anti-metastatic activities. Bioinformatics, molecular docking, and experimental studies to dissect the molecular mechanism of anti-migratory activity revealed that withanone, withaferin A, and withanone–withaferin A target mortalin and hnRNP-K proteins involved in metastasis and angiogenesis.

- Computational methods are often used to gain insight into how compounds work at the molecular level. Such analyses often help to reduce the cost of expensive experiments and drug development. Withaferin A and withanone bind to the mortalin–p53 protein complex, stopping cell growth, and to hnRNP-K and DNA, inhibiting the migration of cancer cells.
- Several clinical studies have shown that Ashwagandha extracts are well tolerated. High doses of 2.0–4.0 grams daily do not result in any significant negative side effects in humans. However, due to variations in raw material composition and extraction methods, high quality and standardization are essential to minimize side effects (Figure 5.1).

In contrast to withaferin A, withanone has less potent anti-cancer activity. At the same time, it has mild effects on normal cells, reflecting its selective toxicity to cancer cells. Normal cells live longer in the presence of low doses of withanone (Figure 5.2), with less accumulation of molecular damage. Some data suggest that withanone has anti-aging activity, which may mean that it also has anti-stress potential.

Modern lifestyles are heavily dependent on chemicals in the form of food, agriculture, cosmetics, textiles, and medical products. As chemical toxicity has become a concern for human health, there is an urgent need for alternative non-toxic natural products. Methoxyacetic acid is a major toxic substance of ester phthalates, which are commonly used as gelling, viscosity, and stabilizing reagents. We investigated the effects of Ashwagandha leaf extract on methoxyacetic acid-induced toxicity in cultured human cells. This chemical causes premature senescence in normal human cells by inducing oxidative stress and DNA and mitochondrial damage. In contrast, treatment with withanone protects cells from these effects. Remarkably, normal cultured cells grown with withanone have a longer lifespan due to reduced molecular

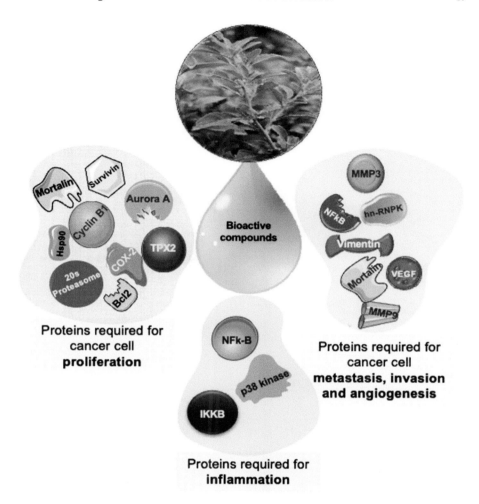

FIGURE 5.1 Proteins involved in the anti-cancer activity of Ashwagandha constituents (withanone, withaferin A, and triethylene glycol). Experimental evidence for effects on cancer cell proliferation, migration, metastasis, angiogenesis, and inflammation.

damage, protection from oxidative damage, and protein degradation activity that recycles molecular damage in cells (Figure 5.3).

Since oxidative stress and accumulation of molecular damage in normal cells is a hallmark of aging and age-related brain diseases, researchers have used brain-derived cells (glioblastoma and neuroblastoma) to investigate the effects of Ashwagandha alcohol extract, withaferin A, and withanone to protect against oxidative stress. Various biochemical and imaging assays in control and treated cells show that low doses of extract and purified withanone can protect glial cells and neurons from oxidative and glutamate damage and induce cell differentiation. These findings support the potential of Ashwagandha to protect neurons and serve as a supplement for brain health (Figure 5.4).

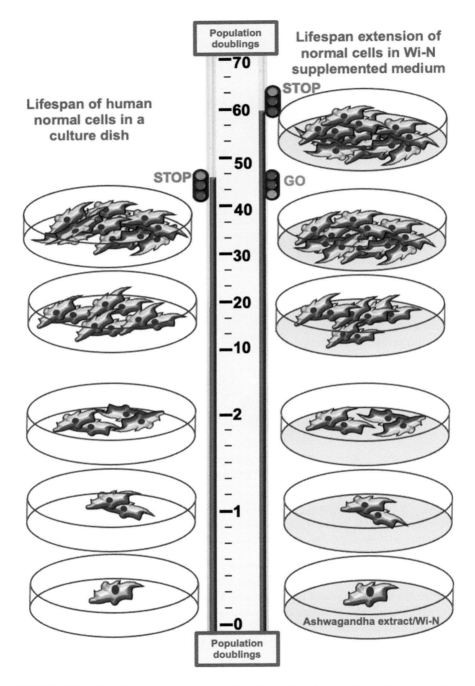

FIGURE 5.2 Graphic representation of the effect of Ashwagandha extract or withanone (Wi-N) on the lifespan of normal human cells. Lifespan extension was reported with Ashwagandha extract rich in Wi-N or Wi-N alone.

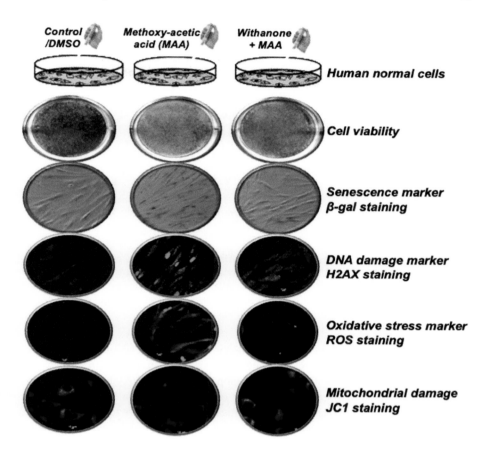

FIGURE 5.3 Pictorial representation of the effect of withanone on cells stressed with toxic chemical (methoxyacetic acid). MAA-exposed cells showed a decrease in cell viability (seen as a decrease in blue staining in the dish), an increase in cells undergoing premature aging (detected by senescence marker-β-gal staining), increase in DNA damage (seen as increase in green staining related to DNA damage marker H2AX), increase in oxidative stress (detected as increase in ROS staining) and increase in mitochondrial damage (seen as decrease in JC1 staining). Cells cultured in MAA+ withanone showed a reversal of all these deleterious changes to a large extent (Priyandoko et al., 2011).

The neuroprotective activity of Ashwagandha alcohol extract and withanone was tested in mouse models of brain injury and recovery. A well-known cholinergic antagonist, scopolamine hydrobromide, was used to induce memory loss in mice. Biochemical analysis revealed that it caused a dose- and time-dependent downregulation of brain-derived neurotrophic factor and glial acidic fibrillary protein expression. Remarkably, mice treated with alcohol extract or withanone show recovery of memory and increased molecular markers of neuronal and glial cell growth, survival, and differentiation. Parallel experiments with cultured human neuroblastoma cells showed reduced activity of neuronal proteins (NF-H, MAP2, PSD-95, GAP-43)

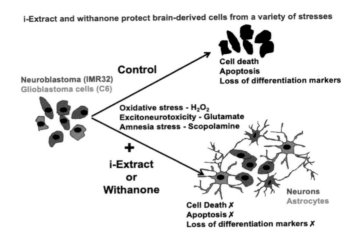

FIGURE 5.4 Schematic representation of the effect of Ashwagandha extract or withanone (Wi-N) on brain-derived cells stressed with oxidative, excitoneurotoxicity, and amnesia stress. Whereas stressed cells showed cell death at large, Ashwagandha extract or withanone supplementation resulted in a significant increase in the number of surviving and differentiated (specialized to perform brain-related functions) cells.

and glial proteins (GFAP) in a model of injury. Remarkably, recovery of these proteins was observed when cells were treated with alcohol extract or withanone.

Memory loss is one of the most common symptoms of Alzheimer's disease. Impressed by the neuroprotective activity of Ashwagandha alcohol extract, the researchers set out to determine its mechanism of action. They tested whether the alcohol extract primarily targets acetylcholine receptors, which regulate memory processes. They reported that the reduction of kallikrein 8 (KLK8) protein, which is involved in learning and memory, was remarkably reversed in mice fed alcohol extract in both the cerebral cortex and hippocampus regions of the brain. Similarly, treatment of a mouse model of Parkinson's disease with alcohol extract improves walking and grooming activities.

Several studies have provided convincing evidence that the leaves of Ashwagandha contain considerable bioactive compounds with anti-cancer activity. These can be concentrated or extracted as alcohol or aqueous extracts with different compositions and activities. High concentrations of withanolides (withaferin A and withanone) stop the growth or cause the death of cancer cells by activating tumor suppressor proteins and inhibiting oncoproteins, while low doses provide anti-stress and rejuvenation by restoring normal cell functions. Since the accumulation of damage caused by chronic stress has been linked to the incidence and severity of cancer, it can be predicted that low doses with anti-stress activity will also have cancer-preventive activity (Figure 5.5).

Aging is closely associated with stress, so these bioactive compounds could be recruited for healthy aging, where one would hope to maintain normal bodily functions over time. The ability to differentiate, which determines specific cell and tissue functions, declines with stress and aging, and reagents or conditions that support

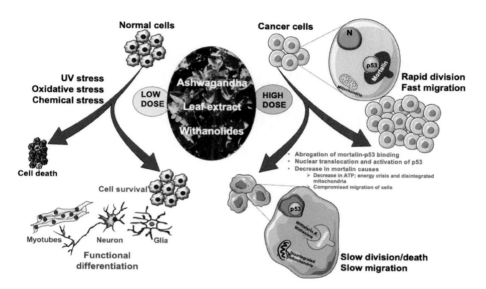

FIGURE 5.5 Schematic representation of the effects of low and high doses of Ashwagandha extract. Low doses protect normal cells from a variety of stresses and cause them to differentiate to perform specific functions. High doses, on the contrary, caused the death of cancer cells by blocking the interaction of mortalin–p53 and thus the activation of p53.

and maintain differentiation are considered health-supporting or health-enhancing. Remarkably, low doses of Ashwagandha leaf extracts, withanone, and withaferin A induce differentiation of brain and muscle-derived cells.

In an experimental study to screen anti-stress compounds using cell culture-based assays, cells were challenged with chemical models of oxidative, metal, or hypoxic stress. The recovery of stressed cells cultured in a normal growth medium or in a medium containing various natural compounds (at non-toxic concentrations) was compared. Of the 70 compounds tested, five compounds caused better recovery of cells subjected to three types of stress. Of note, these five compounds included withaferin A, methoxy withaferin A, withanone, triethylene glycol, and Ashwagandha leaf extract. Through extensive molecular assays, it was found that while stressed cells accumulate oxidative stress, DNA damage, mitochondrial abnormalities, and protein aggregates, these compounds caused significant protection against such damage. Since these abnormalities are common in aging cells, normal human cells at young, mature, and senescent stages, representing different levels of stress accumulation, were exposed to these compounds. Remarkably, withanone, triethylene glycol, and their mixture-treated pre-senescent and senescent cells showed an increase in viability and proliferation compared to the matched control cells, suggesting (i) the anti-stress potential of these compounds and (ii) their use in the treatment of age- and environmental stress-related pathologies.

6 Does Ashwagandha Have Any Effect on the Prevention and Treatment of COVID-19?

A novel coronavirus, SARS-CoV-2 (Severe Acute Respiratory Syndrome CoronaVirus-2), emerged in Wuhan, China, in December 2019 and spread rapidly around the world through human-to-human transmission, causing the COVID-19 pandemic. In less than half a year, ~5 million people were infected with ~0.5 million reported deaths, declaring a global health emergency. The high number of infections and deaths prompted the urgent initiation of new lines of drug and vaccine development, on the one hand, and the repurposing of existing drugs and traditional home remedies, on the other.

Coronaviruses (family Coronaviridae; order Nidovirales) are large, enveloped, positive-stranded RNA viruses. Their name comes from their corona-like appearance under the microscope. SARS-CoV-2 is an enveloped, single-stranded RNA β-coronavirus similar to the viruses that cause Severe Acute Respiratory Syndrome (SARS) and Middle East Respiratory Syndrome. SARS-CoV-2 is also closely related to two other SARS-like coronaviruses from bats (CoVZC45 and bat-SL-CoVZXC21). The coronavirus genome is the largest of all RNA viruses and is packaged in a helical shell consisting of a nucleocapsid protein surrounded by an envelope consisting of three structural proteins: membrane protein, envelope protein, and spike protein. The membrane and envelope proteins are involved in virus assembly, and the spike protein (which forms the spike-like protrusions from the surface of the virus, giving it a crown-like appearance) mediates its entry into host cells. The virus enters the respiratory tract through the nose or mouth. After an incubation period of approximately 3–7 days, the virus causes symptoms of common cold/bronchitis (sneezing, nasal congestion, runny nose, cough, headache, fever, pneumonia, asthenia, and airway inflammation) in birds and mammals. In contrast to animals, where the virus infects multiple tissues and causes multiple diseases, in humans, the virus causes primarily respiratory infections with mild cold-like symptoms and occasional gastrointestinal symptoms. Infected individuals shed the virus in nasal secretions and mucous membranes, resulting in disease transmission that can often be at least partially controlled by good hygiene.

DOI: 10.1201/9781032705743-6

The entry of SARS-CoV-2 into the host cell depends on the interaction of the virus with a cell surface protein receptor called ACE-2. ACE-2 is a membrane protein expressed primarily in the lung, kidney, intestine, and heart. It contains two sites to which the S protein of the SARS-CoV virus binds. Mutations surrounding these sites on ACE2 affect the infectivity of the virus and the pathogenesis of the disease. SARS-CoV-2 has a higher binding affinity for ACE2 than other strains of SARS-CoV. After binding to the ACE-2 receptor, the viral spike protein fuses with the membrane of the host cell. This process is facilitated by another cell membrane protein called transmembrane protease serine 2 (TMPRSS-2). ACE-2 and TMPRSS-2 act as gates for SARS-CoV-2 entry into host cells. The proteins thus regulate how well the virus can infect cells and spread. Host cells enriched in TMPRSS2 proteins are highly susceptible to SARS-CoV-2 infection, and inhibitors of TMPRSS2 reduce infection and the severity of disease symptoms. Once inside the host cell, the virus uses the host cell's resources to decode viral genetic information into proteins and produce more viruses to infect neighboring cells – continuing the cycle of rapid, high replication. Because of TMPRSS2's critical role in viral infection, protease inhibitors (which block TMPRSS2 activity) are considered potential drugs to treat and prevent viral infections. Camostat mesylate, a protease inhibitor used clinically to treat chronic pancreatitis, was shown to partially suppress SARS-CoV-2 infection. Upon entry into the host cell, the SARS-CoV-2 virus replicase gene encodes two polyproteins, ppla and pplab, which are processed into their functional forms by a viral protein called the major protease (M^{pro}, also known as 3C-like protease). M^{pro} is essential for the proliferation and infection cycle of the virus, making it an attractive target for anti-viral drugs.

In the absence of drugs and vaccines for SARS-CoV-2, several studies have used computational approaches to explore the repurposing of existing drugs to find immediate therapeutic candidates for COVID-19. Most of these studies targeted (i) viral proteins including proteases, spike glycoprotein, RNA polymerase, nucleocapsid, and envelope proteins, and (ii) human cell surface receptors ACE-2 and TMPRSS-2. Ashwagandha is believed to be an immunity enhancer and has a variety of prophylactic and therapeutic activities. Several studies have provided evidence for its antimicrobial activities discussed earlier in this book. Withaferin A also has inhibitory activity against human papillomavirus and influenza viruses. To this end, we tested the active withanolides of Ashwagandha (withaferin A and withanone) for their ability to bind to a highly conserved viral protein, Mpro, which is essential for viral replication and survival. Withanone, but not withaferin A, showed strong binding to Mpro with a binding energy equivalent to a known M^{pro} inhibitor (N3), predicting that Wi-N may serve as a natural drug for COVID-19. We also investigated the potential of withaferin A and withanone to bind to TMPRSS2 and found that although both withaferin A and withanone could bind and stably interact with TMPRSS2, withanone showed stronger binding (Figure 6.1). Not only that, human cells treated with

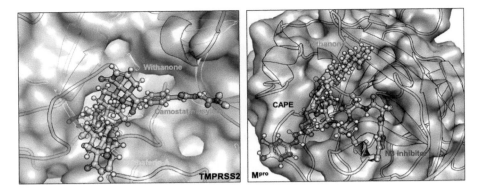

FIGURE 6.1   Surface view of the cell surface protein TMPRSS-2 showing binding of witha-ferin A (Wi-A), withanone (Wi-N), and camostat mesylate (a known inhibitor of TMPRSS2) at its catalytic site (left) and the viral M^{pro} protein showing binding of its known inhibitor (N3) and withanone at the same region (right).

withanone showed a lower level of expression of TMPRSS2, predicting three-way action of withanone to deal with SARS-CoV-2 (blocking its entry into host cells by interacting with TMPRSS2, downregulating TMPRSS2 expression and decreasing viral survival by inhibiting viral M^{pro} protein).

Similarly, in extended studies, the efficacy of eight Ashwagandha withanolides was tested against ACE2 and TMPRSS2 receptors and it was found that (i) most of these made stable interactions with these proteins and (ii) four withanolides, with-aferin A, withanone, withanoside IV and withanoside V caused significant reduc-tion in their mRNA and protein expression. Based on these, Ashwagandha extracts containing a mixture of withanolides were considered useful and validated in cell culture-based experiments, suggesting that Ashwagandha is a useful resource for COVID-19 treatment (Figure 6.2).

Experimental assays were carried out to validate the anti-viral activity of withanolides. Using the SARS-CoV-2 replication assay, it was found that several withanolides caused a decrease in the expression of the viral envelope (E-gene) and nucleocapsid sequences (N-gene), which indicates their potential to inhibit virus replication. Remdesivir, a clini-cally used anti-viral drug, was used as a positive control and showed 68%–99% inhibi-tion of virus replication in a dose-dependent manner. Cells treated with withanolides derived from Ashwagandha, such as withanone, withanolide B, and withanoside V,

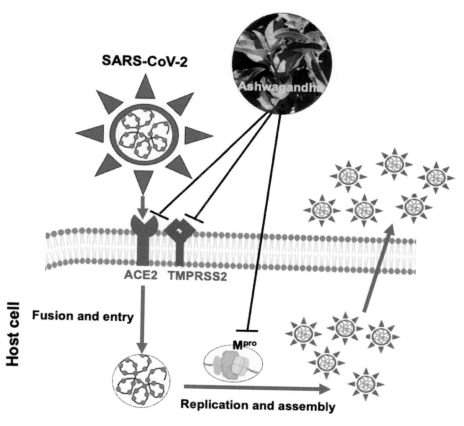

FIGURE 6.2 Schematic representation of host cell membrane proteins and SARS-CoV-2 viral proteins targeted by Ashwagandha. Inhibition of host cell surface proteins (TMPRSS2 and ACE2) required for viral entry into cells and inhibition of viral protein (M^pro) required for viral division in cells were reported.

showed an average of ~66%, 84%, and 73% inhibition, respectively. However, withanolide A, withanoside IV, and 12-deoxywithastramonolide caused less than 50% inhibition. These studies have supported the anti-COVID-19 activity of Ashwagandha withanolides and more of the extracts possessing a mixture of these compounds.

7 What Next?

Signature Compounds and Their Corresponding Activities as Well as the Importance of Quality and Chemotyping

The combination of a long history of use in Ayurveda and modern research strongly supports moving Ashwagandha out of the laboratory. The next step is to prepare Ashwagandha for wider use in society in a more precise, safe, and secure manner. However, there are still hurdles to overcome for production and commercialization. These include seasonal and regional variations in the bioactive component of the plant material, quality control, and defining the exact chemical composition of the plant, known as chemotype. Certain soil factors (including microbiota and physical and chemical factors) significantly influence plant growth and characteristics. These variables can have a significant impact on the amount of active ingredients or toxicants in a plant. For this reason, the monitoring of soil, plant growth, and plant parts containing bioactive compounds requires special attention and expertise. It is particularly important to avoid metal and microbial contamination.

Traditional Ashwagandha cultivation is limited by poor seed viability and germination, low yield, and inconsistent production of secondary metabolites. Pest and pathogen infestation is also a major challenge in Ashwagandha cultivation. Recently, global climate change and unethical agricultural practices have become major concerns as these factors can stress plants and affect their growth and development. Some studies on the influence of heavy metal stress on Ashwagandha report that copper toxicity reduces fresh plant weight, chlorophyll content, and carotenoid content. As a result, these plants have shorter roots and shoots. Biochemical analysis also shows increased lipid peroxidation and oxidative stress levels. Biotechnological approaches using organ, tissue, and cell culture offer alternative and modern solutions. Plant propagation in the laboratory helps to rapidly multiply selected cultivars to produce high-quality plants. Genetic manipulation and secondary metabolite engineering hold great promise for improving secondary metabolites and overall crop improvement. To address all of these concerns, scientists have developed methods to produce Ashwagandha indoors under controlled environments and growing conditions. One such method is described below.

DOI: 10.1201/9781032705743-7

7.1 ACTIVE INGREDIENT–ENRICHED HYDROPONIC ASHWAGANDHA

Hydroponics, the technique of growing plants in water, takes advantage of the fact that plants can synthesize all the nutrients they need from inorganic ions, water, carbon dioxide, and artificial light. It provides a convenient way to (i) avoid unpredictable extreme weather conditions that affect growing plants in soil, (ii) protect against environmental stresses including industrial pollutants and pesticides, and (iii) ensure stable levels of active compounds that are important for the plant's value as functional foods or medicines. Hydroponics is particularly important for seasonal plants and functional foods to provide stable and controlled nutrient resources.

Ashwagandha leaves contain higher levels of the active withanolide compounds withaferin A and withanone than the plant's roots. These compounds are useful for disease therapy and improving quality of life. The hydroponic cultivation of Ashwagandha has been explored to produce high-quality plants enriched with active ingredients. A plant factory in Saitama, Japan, established the process by designing layered hydroponic growing chambers with a large growing area. These chambers supplied temperature-controlled air using: (i) temperature-controlled heat-insulated panels, (ii) high-precision air conditioning and air ducting systems for airflow, and (iii) automated ultrasonic humidifiers for moisture control. Carbon dioxide (CO_2) concentration was monitored by sensors and supplied in liquid form. The nutrient solution was circulated by a pump to optimize and automate its concentration. Nutrients were supplied by a specific fertilizer mix that was automatically maintained at specific concentrations monitored by electrodes. Hybrid electrode fluorescent lamps exposed the plants to four different wavelengths of light, including fluorescent, red, red:blue, and red:blue:green.

The factory also studied the effect of various environmental conditions – such as UV light, temperature, pH, and nutrients – on plant characteristics, including plant height, number of leaves, and weight of shoots and roots. The results showed that Ashwagandha could be successfully grown in a hydroponic facility. In addition, UV-stressed plants showed high levels of anti-cancer activity, suggesting the possibility of growing plants enriched with specific compounds. For example, the leaves of plants grown under red light had ten times more withanone than withaferin A, and the leaves of plants grown under UV light had high levels of withaferin A. Remarkably, a mixture of red, blue, and green light showed high levels of both withanone and withaferin A (Figure 7.1).

Often, a variety of plant biotechnologies have been used to study the function of genes, understand their regulation, and increase the levels of secondary metabolites. In this premise, it was found that transgenic hairy root cultures produce and easily maintain large biomass and increase the level and rate of synthesis of Ashwagandha secondary metabolites, including withanolide A, withanolide D, and withaferin A. To enhance the commercial value of Ashwagandha, researchers have considered breeding stress-tolerant and disease-resistant cultivars of Ashwagandha. Among various diseases, leaf spot (characterized by brownish to black spots on the leaves) is one of the most common diseases. It is caused by a fungus (*Alternaria alternata*)

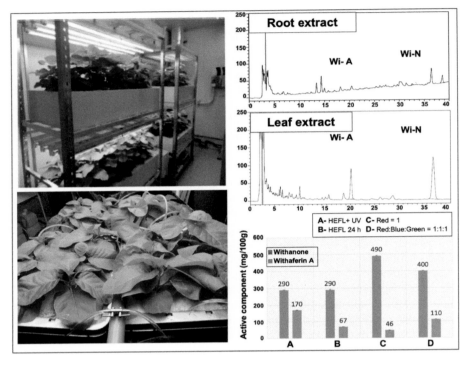

FIGURE 7.1 Images showing hydroponic cultivation of Ashwagandha (left) and quantification of active compounds in hydroponically grown plants. The leaf extract has a higher level of bioactive withanolides than the root extract (right-top), and it is possible to modulate the number of active compounds by exposing the plants to different types of light (red/blue/green) (Kaul et al., 2016).

that degrades pharmaceutically important secondary metabolites. Ongoing efforts are underway in many laboratories to develop a sensitive detection system for fungal infection, disease-related proteins, and disease-resistant cultivars.

Chemical fertilizers often used to increase crop yields, not only affect the quality of the plants but can also alter their levels of active compounds. For Ashwagandha,

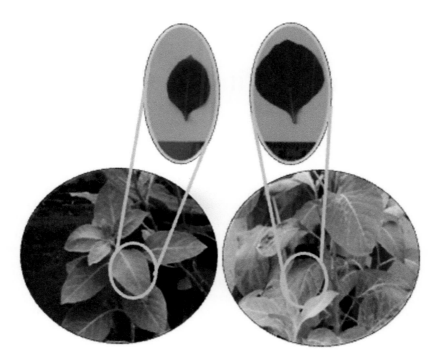

FIGURE 7.2 Biomass of Ashwagandha was increased by cultivation in vermicompost. A significant increase in leaf size was reported.

researchers have adopted vermicompost (made by earthworms) as the organic fertilizer of choice. Pre-soaking Ashwagandha seeds in vermicompost mixes improve their germination (Figure 7.2). A combination of pre-soaking seeds and growing in vermicompost further improves both germination and seedling growth. Plants grown in the presence of vermicompost have higher leaf and root mass and earlier onset of flowering and fruiting. In addition, the leaves of plants grown in vermicompost have higher levels of the active withanolides withanone, withanolide A, and withaferin A. Such methods can serve as a simple and inexpensive method to improve the yield and pharmaceutical components of Ashwagandha leaves.

8 Collection of True Stories and Testimonials

8.1 ASHWAGANDHA CALMED ME DOWN

I have been dealing with chronic anxiety for 16 years. It invaded my daily life, my job, my relationships, my confidence, my sleep, and my health. It was truly exhausting. Desperate for a remedy, I read about the adaptogenic effects of Ashwagandha. I was skeptical about the wonders it claimed to do, but I wanted to try it anyway. I decided to try it, and it did indeed work wonders for me. I took two capsules in the morning and two just before bed. Sometimes I would add a teaspoon to my green smoothie or green tea. Within a few weeks, I was breathing easier, feeling much calmer, sleeping better, and my relationships with others began to improve. I was motivated to continue on the same dosage. Three months later, I feel pretty normal. Normally, one would take lorazepam or imipramine (the generics of Ativan and Tofranil) for anxiety, but the power of the Ashwagandha leaf worked better for me. It lowered cortisol (stress chemical released in our bodies) and got rid of my insomnia. My family's health has improved – that means a lot! (Figure 8.1).

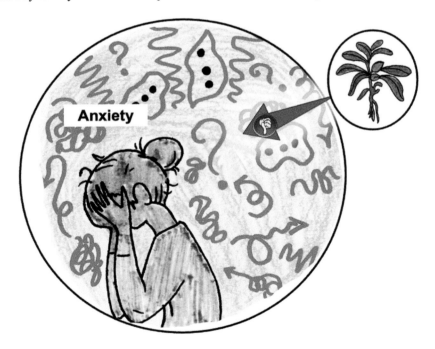

FIGURE 8.1

DOI: 10.1201/9781032705743-8

8.2 ASHWAGANDHA HAS IMPROVED MY FATIGUE

I am a person who does not like to take medicines. I think it's not good for my body and has strange effects. Suddenly, at the age of 45, I felt no energy; I was suggested to take multivitamins, minerals, proteins, and many more. I tried to change my diet, but it did not work. Feeling depressed and tired, I came across Ashwagandha as an energizing and calming substance. After taking it for 2 weeks, I felt that it gave a kind of balance to my stressed body. I am able to handle my work, stress, anxiety, and fatigue much better (Figure 8.2).

8.3 ASHWAGANDHA CURED MY EPILEPSY

Unfortunately, I had my first epileptic seizure when I was just 18 years old and preparing for my high school exams. One day, I suddenly fell to the ground in a violent seizure, shocking my whole family. My doctor told me that I had epilepsy. Obviously, my parents were very worried about my future (education, marriage, etc.).

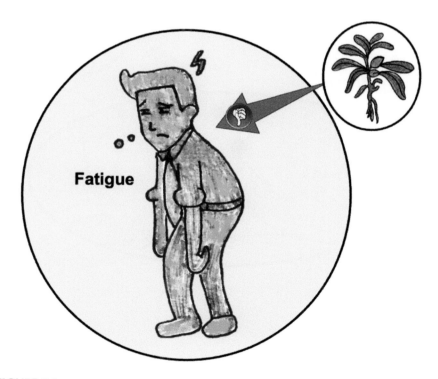

FIGURE 8.2

I was told that treatment for epilepsy includes surgery, vagal nerve stimulation, a ketogenic diet, transcranial magnetic stimulation, and other alternative/complementary therapies such as yoga, aerobic exercise, music therapy, acupuncture, and herbal remedies. These therapies relax the body and mind and reduce stress, which helps to improve seizure control in most cases. Most patients choose alternative therapies because anti-epileptic drugs have unpleasant side effects, require long-term treatment, and often fail. I studied a lot of information on the Internet about calming herbs and decided to try Ashwagandha leaf powder. It worked for me. Since I started taking it, I feel much calmer and less anxious – much less frequent headaches and almost no epileptic seizures for the past 2 years (Figure 8.3).

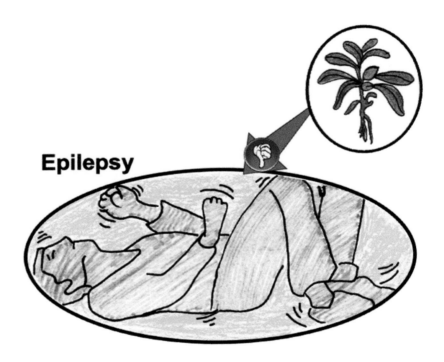

FIGURE 8.3

8.4 ASHWAGANDHA REDUCED MY PARKINSON'S TREMORS

I am a high-level professional with a history of leading highly skilled teams in a transportation company. Suddenly, at the age of 45, I felt that my activity was being restricted and I started having tremors in my arms. I was diagnosed with early-onset Parkinson's disease, which was a huge shock. Thanks to my friend who introduced me to Ashwagandha. Since then – more than 6 years now – I have been taking Ashwagandha and am happily living my normal life and meeting the challenges of work without much difficulty. I owe my normal life to Ashwagandha (Figure 8.4).

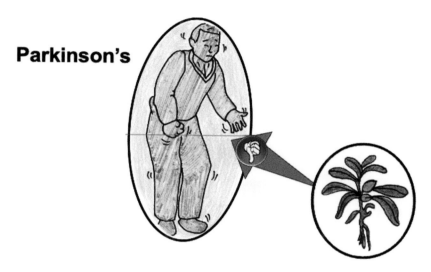

Parkinson's

FIGURE 8.4

8.5 ASHWAGANDHA EASED MY KNEE PAIN

I am 70 years old and have had a healthy life with minor issues of blood pressure and diabetes that required mild medication. I lead a house-in life with very little outside exposure. I do not exercise or walk daily. All I do is cook for the family, watch TV, and pass the time doing housework. Well, I knew that this was not the best healthy life, and, besides, I love to eat fried and good food. About 5–7 years ago, my knees started refusing to cope with my lifestyle. Painkillers and anti-inflammatories were the only remedies, and I became dependent on them regularly. Some time ago, I started taking glucosamine and Ashwagandha leaf powder and was surprised to find that I needed much fewer painkillers and anti-inflammatory pills. I have started to sleep well and feel calm and serene. I want to go out and interact with people (Figure 8.5).

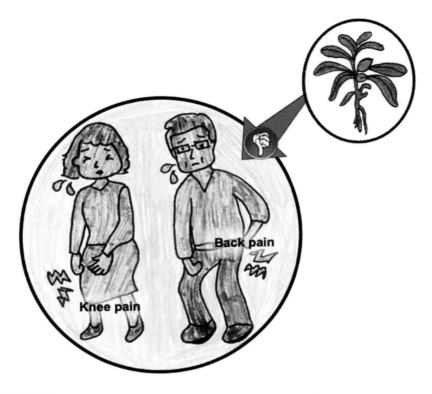

FIGURE 8.5

8.6   ASHWAGANDHA WORKED FOR MY DIABETES

At the age of 59 and just a few months before I officially retired from my job, when I was feeling depressed, I discovered that I had diabetes. Although it was not too bad, the doctor asked me to control my sugar intake and prescribed a medicine to take every morning. I have been on this regimen for the past 3 years. Knowing that Ashwagandha improves diabetes in laboratory studies, I started taking it. Two weeks later, my blood sugar levels returned to normal. I have been taking Ashwagandha regularly and have been able to reduce my prescribed diabetes medication to half a tablet instead of one. I feel happy about it (Figure 8.6).

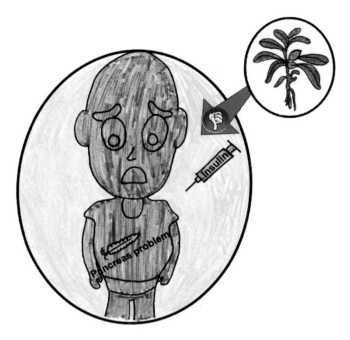

FIGURE 8.6

8.7 ASHWAGANDHA CURED MY NON-HODGKIN'S LYMPHOMA

I have tried every modern medicine offered for my disease, non-Hodgkin's lymphoma. Most of these drugs caused additional complications, including worsening diabetes, infections, depression, and ulcers in my throat. I was unable to eat. After a year of struggling unsuccessfully with painkillers and anti-depressants, I decided to try Ashwagandha. Miracles do happen – I believed it and I saw it! After a short time on Ashwagandha, my throat ulcers receded, I felt better, and I was able to cut my steroid dose in half. A month later, my blood test showed a remarkable improvement in my white blood cell count, and inflammation and infections began to disappear. Three months later, I stopped the steroids completely and returned to my normal life with a healthy weight and state of mind. I am completely cured and enjoying my professional and personal life again (Figure 8.7).

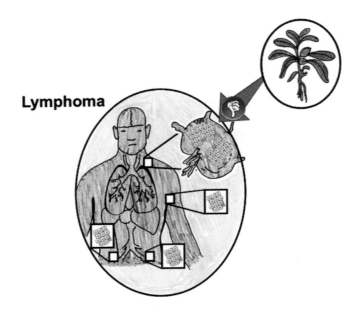

FIGURE 8.7

8.8   ASHWAGANDHA HELPED ME GET RID OF MY BURNING SENSATION POST-RADIATION TREATMENT OF PROSTATE CANCER

I was diagnosed with prostate cancer and had to go through a few cycles of chemo- and radiotherapy. It was hard enough having to go through sickness, vomiting, and stomach upset issues. The worst was the after-effects of radiotherapy that raised a continuous burning sensation in my body. I could not eat or sleep well. I just happened to get information on the good and calming effects of Ashwagandha and tried

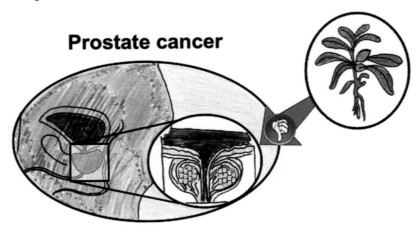

FIGURE 8.8

it. I started taking the leaf powder regularly and the burning sensation disappeared in about 8–10 days. I was also able to sleep well in a few days. Ever since, I have continued taking Ashwagadha twice a day. It has been more than 5 years and am doing well. Thanks to Ashwagandha! (Figure 8.8).

8.9 ASHWAGANDHA HELPED TO TREAT MY LUNG CANCER

At the age of 70, a routine chest X-ray revealed a small lump in my left lung. Unfortunately, further tests proved it to be malignant lung cancer. I started taking Ashwagandha leaf powder before any prescribed medication. I went through the first line of targeted oral therapy without much difficulty (except that it is expensive and hard to afford). It worked to reduce my tumor to 80% in half a year. However, it stopped working and I was switched to a second line of drugs after 15 months, followed by radiation therapy after the next ~12 months. I have trusted and kept my company with Ashwagandha all the way through, and I take 7.5 g of leaf powder every day. My tumor has not metastasized to other tissues. I feel that Ashwagandha has acted as a great buffer that has made my journey through a difficult time with lung cancer easier. Every conventional drug I took showed effects for a longer period than expected. I was afraid of the radiation, but it was not as strong as I thought – I credit that to the Ashwagandha leaf powder. Now I have my appetite and physical strength back to normal for my age and I stay calm and strong (Figure 8.9).

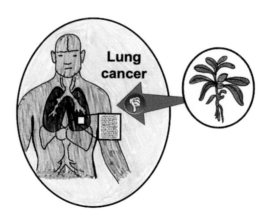

FIGURE 8.9

8.10   ASHWAGANDHA IS HELPING ME WITH BREAST CANCER

I was diagnosed with ovarian cancer at age 47. After getting various chemo and other devastating treatments, I recovered and started my normal life. Unfortunately, breast cancer was diagnosed after 20 years. Age factor and my earlier experience with chemotherapy was quite terrifying. There was no choice but to go through another set of chemos and surgery. Looking for alternative treatments was a reasonable consideration after the successful first line of treatment. I chose to try Ashwagandha after discussing it with some experts and ayurvedic specialists. It has been 12 years since I have taken 300 mg of leaf powder twice a day. I keep my normal energy and powder for day-to-day work. No big issues with general cold or infections. Cancers have not come back as yet, and I have confidence in this miraculous herb (Figure 8.10).

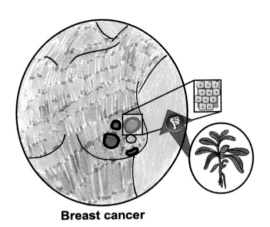

Breast cancer

FIGURE 8.10

8.11   ASHWAGANDHA HELPS ME MANAGE HAILEY'S DISEASE

Hailey's disease, also known as familial benign chronic pemphigus, is a skin disease that is common in middle-aged and elderly people and is very difficult to cure. Blisters repeatedly appear in the armpits, crotch, around the anus, under the breasts, and in high-friction, soft, and moist areas during high temperatures and humid seasons. These are often accompanied by infectious diseases. It is a hereditary disease caused by a mutation of the gene called ATP2C1. In most cases, people do not know the onset of the disease but remain worried when a family member has it. It is very difficult to cure, so it is important to start treatment as early as possible and before blisters appear. The worst part is that it becomes difficult to heal with repeated recurrences, as the skin becomes moist, hypertrophic, itchy, erosive, and painful. Summer heat, humidity, and secondary infection make it terrible with an unbearable burning sensation. The worst ones also get pus/exudate and a foul odor. I know there is no basic cure, so I have to rely on anti-rash corticosteroid anti-inflammatory drugs.

Maintenance of symptomatic treatment and management of the remission state is the best. I learned that Ashwagandha is an anti-stress herb, and I started taking it without really expecting any effects on my Hailey's disease. I started taking half a teaspoon in hot water, just like green tea, twice a day. It has worked dramatically for me. My life has changed. I would recommend it to anyone with Hailey's disease (Figure 8.11).

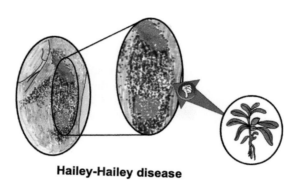

Hailey-Hailey disease

FIGURE 8.11

Final Thoughts

Ashwagandha is known as the queen of Ayurveda and Indian ginseng for its health benefits. In traditional Indian home medicine, Ashwagandha has been used to treat various ailments ranging from the common cold to arthritis, brain abnormalities, and cancer. Prescribed as a general tonic to improve overall health and trusted for its miraculous effects, its use dates back nearly 5,000 years – passed down through generations as "wisdom of the mouth" for various disease prevention and therapeutic activities. It is included in the GRAS (generally recorded as safe) category of herbs under sections 201(s) and 409 of the Federal Food, Drug, and Cosmetic Act, and therefore clinical trials for its trusted therapeutic effects were long considered unnecessary. Only in recent years have experimental studies using cultured human cells and animal models begun to test the bioactivities of Ashwagandha extracts.

This book presents not only the bioactivities and experimental evidence of Ashwagandha but also the mechanism of action of its active constituents. Withanolides (withaferin A, withanone, and withanolide A) are considered to be the major bioactive compounds in Ashwagandha. Their levels vary in different parts of the plant, geographical locations, and harvesting seasons. Laboratory studies have shown that, although these withanolides are closely related in structure, they differ in their behavior and bioactivity and thus have different functions.

Withaferin A is mainly found in the leaves and has remarkable anti-cancer activities. Withanone has milder activity, while the methoxy derivative of withaferin A has no anti-cancer activity at all. Cell culture–based experiments, in which knockdown of proteins can be easily recruited, revealed different pathways through which these anti-cancer activities act. It was found that these anti-cancer components of Ashwagandha work through multiple pathways, including the activation of tumor suppressor proteins (proteins that cause cells to stop growing and divide uncontrollably) and inactivation of oncogenes (that allow cells to continue to proliferate uncontrollably), which collectively stop the growth or cause the death of cancer cells. Withaferin A inhibits the proliferation of cancer cells with activated telomerase or other alternative mechanisms of telomere elongation, strongly suggesting its potential for drug development (especially for cancers that do not respond to telomerase-inhibiting drugs). Remarkably, some extract components, including withanone or the methoxy derivative of withaferin A, protect normal cells against chemical-induced toxicity and other stresses. These data convincingly predict that an Ashwagandha extract with a mixture of "toxic" and "non-toxic and protective" components is the best choice (Figure 1). This strategy may even turn the negative side effects usually associated with chemotherapy into benefits. We hope that this book will serve as a

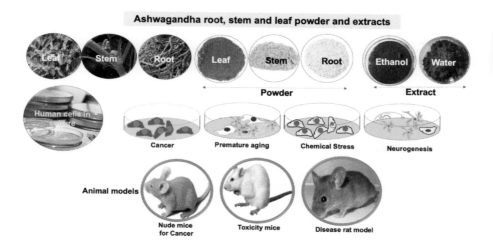

FIGURE 1 Diagram depicting our study models: Bioactivities in leaf, stem, and root extracts were investigated using cellular models for cancer, premature aging, chemical stresses, and neurogenesis. Rodent disease models were also utilized as needed.

guide for people who use or wish to use Ashwagandha. Advice from a doctor for the purpose of its use and dose is highly recommended. We wish all of you good health with Ashwagandha.

Selected Readings

Abeesh, P., Guruvayoorappan, C. The therapeutic effects of withaferin a against cancer: Overview and updates. *Curr Mol Med* 2023. doi:10.2174/1566524023666230418094 708.

Alanazi, H.H., Elfaki, E. The immunomodulatory role of *Withania somnifera* (L.) dunal in inflammatory diseases. *Front Pharmacol* 2023, 14: 1084757. doi:10.3389/fphar.2023.1084757.

Bashir, A., Nabi, M., Tabassum, N., Afzal, S., Ayoub, M. An updated review on phytochemistry and molecular targets of *Withania somnifera* (L.) *Dunal* (Ashwagandha). *Front Pharmacol* 2023, 14: 1049334. doi:10.3389/fphar.2023.1049334.

Chaudhary, A., Kalra, R.S., Malik, V., Katiyar, S.P., Sundar, D., Kaul, S.C., Wadhwa, R. 2, 3-dihydro-3beta-methoxy withaferin: A lacks anti-metastasis potency: Bioinformatics and experimental evidences. *Sci Rep* 2019, 9: 17344. doi:10.1038/s41598-019-53568-6.

Dhanjal, J.K., Kumar, V., Garg, S., Subramani, C., Agarwal, S., Wang, J., Zhang, H., Kaul, A., Kalra, R.S., Kaul, S.C., Vrati, S., Sundar, D., Wadhwa, R. Molecular mechanism of anti-SARS-CoV2 activity of Ashwagandha-derived withanolides. *Int J Biol Macromol* 2021, 184: 297–312. doi:10.1016/j.ijbiomac.2021.06.015.

Dutta, R., Khalil, R., Green, R., Mohapatra, S.S., Mohapatra, S. *Withania Somnifera* (Ashwagandha) and withaferin A: Potential in integrative oncology. *Int J Mol Sci* 2019, 20: doi:10.3390/ijms20215310.

Gao, R., Shah, N., Lee, J.S., Katiyar, S.P., Li, L., Oh, E., Sundar, D., Yun, C.O., Kaul, S.C., Wadhwa, R. Withanone rich combination of Ashwagandha withanolides restricts metastasis and angiogenesis through hnRNP-K. *Mol Cancer Ther* 2014, 13: 2930–2940. doi:10.1158/1535-7163.MCT-14-0324.

Gaurav, H., Yadav, D., Maurya, A., Yadav, H., Yadav, R., Shukla, A.C., Sharma, M., Gupta, V.K., Palazon, J. Biodiversity, biochemical profiling, and pharmaco-commercial applications of Withania somnifera: A review. *Molecules* 2023, 28. doi:10.3390/molecules28031208.

Gautam, A., Wadhwa, R., Thakur, M.K. Involvement of hippocampal Arc in amnesia and its recovery by alcoholic extract of Ashwagandha leaves. *Neurobiol Learn Mem* 2013, 106: 177–184. doi:10.1016/j.nlm.2013.08.009.

Gautam, A., Wadhwa, R., Thakur, M.K. Assessment of cholinergic properties of ashwagandha leaf-extract in the amnesic mouse brain. *Ann Neurosci* 2016, 23: 68–75. doi:10.1159/000443573.

Grover, A., Singh, R., Shandilya, A., Priyandoko, D., Agrawal, V., Bisaria, V.S., Wadhwa, R., Kaul, S.C., Sundar, D. Ashwagandha derived withanone targets TPX2-Aurora A complex: Computational and experimental evidence to its anticancer activity. *PLoS One* 2012, 7: e30890. doi:10.1371/journal.pone.0030890.

Kataria, H., Shah, N., Kaul, S.C., Wadhwa, R., Kaur, G. Water extract of ashwagandha leaves limits proliferation and migration, and induces differentiation in glioma cells. *Evid Based Complement Alternat Med* 2011, 267614. doi:10.1093/ecam/nep188.

Kataria, H., Wadhwa, R., Kaul, S.C., Kaur, G. Water extract from the leaves of *Withania somnifera* protect RA differentiated C6 and IMR-32 cells against glutamate-induced excitotoxicity. *PLoS One* 2012, 7: e37080. doi:10.1371/journal.pone.0037080.

Kataria, H., Wadhwa, R., Kaul, S.C., Kaur, G. *Withania somnifera* water extract as a potential candidate for differentiation based therapy of human neuroblastomas. *PLoS One* 2013, 8: e55316. doi:10.1371/journal.pone.0055316.

Kalra, R.S., Kumar, V., Dhanjal, J.K., Garg, S., Li, X., Kaul, S.C., Sundar, D., Wadhwa, R. COVID19-inhibitory activity of withanolides involves targeting of the host cell surface receptor ACE2: Insights from computational and biochemical assays. *J Biomol Struct Dyn* 2022, 40: 7885–7898. doi:10.1080/07391102.2021.1902858.

Kaul, S. C., Ishida, Y., Tamura, K., Wada, T., Iitsuka, T., Garg, S., Kim, M., Gao, R., Nakai, S., Okamoto, Y., Terao, K., Wadhwa R. Novel methods to generate active ingredients-enriched Ashwagandha leaves and extracts. *PLoS One* 2016, 11: e0166945. doi:10.1371/journal.pone.0166945.21.

Kaul, S. C., Wadhwa R. *Science of Ashwagandha: Preventive and Therapeutic Potentials*, Springer, 2017

Kaur K., Rani, G., Widodo, N., Nagpal, A., Taira, K., Kaul, S.C., Wadhwa, R. Evaluation of the anti-proliferative and anti-oxidative activities of leaf extract from in vivo and in vitro raised Ashwagandha. *Food Chem Toxicol* 2004, 42: 2015–2020. doi:10.1016/j.fct.2004.07.015.

Kaur, A., Singh, B., Ohri, P., Wang, J., Wadhwa, R., Kaul, S. C., Pati, P. K., Kaur, A. Organic cultivation of Ashwagandha with improved biomass and high content of active withanolides: Use of vermicompost. *PLoS One* 2018, 13: e0194314. doi:10.1371/journal. pone.0194314.

Kaushik, M. K., Kaul, S. C., Wadhwa, R., Yanagisawa, M., Urade, Y. Triethylene glycol, an active component of Ashwagandha (*Withania somnifera*) leaves, is responsible for sleep induction. *PLoS One* 2017, 12: e0172508. doi:10.1371/journal.pone.0172508.

Konar, A., Shah, N., Singh, R., Saxena, N., Kaul, S.C., Wadhwa, R., Thakur, M.K. Protective role of Ashwagandha leaf extract and its component withanone on scopolamine-induced changes in the brain and brain-derived cells. *PLoS One* 2011, 6: e27265. doi:10.1371/journal.pone.0027265.

Konar, A., Gupta, R., Shukla, R.K., Maloney, B., Khanna, V.K., Wadhwa, R., Lahiri, D.K., Thakur, M.K. M1 muscarinic receptor is a key target of neuroprotection, neuroregeneration and memory recovery by i-Extract from *Withania somnifera*. *Sci Rep* 2019, 9: 13990. doi:10.1038/s41598-019-48238-6.

Kuboyama, T., Tohda, C., Komatsu, K. Effects of Ashwagandha (roots of *Withania somnifera*) on neurodegenerative diseases. *Biol Pharm Bull* 2014, 37: 892–897.

Kumar, V., Dhanjal, J.K., Kaul, S.C., Wadhwa, R., Sundar, D. Withanone and caffeic acid phenethyl ester are predicted to interact with main protease (M(pro)) of SARS-CoV-2 and inhibit its activity. *J Biomol Struct Dyn* 2021, 39: 3842–3854. doi:10.1080/07391102.2020.1772108.

Kumar, V., Dhanjal, J.K., Bhargava, P., Kaul, A., Wang, J., Zhang, H., Kaul, S.C., Wadhwa, R., Sundar, D. Withanone and withaferin-A are predicted to interact with transmembrane protease serine 2 (TMPRSS2) and block entry of SARS-CoV-2 into cells. *J Biomol Struct Dyn* 2022, 40: 1–13. doi:10.1080/07391102.2020.1775704.

Macharia, J.M., Kaposztas, Z., Bence, R.L. Medicinal characteristics of Withania somnifera L. in colorectal cancer management. *Pharmaceuticals (Basel)* 2023, 16: doi:10.3390/ph16070915.

Malik, V., Kumar, V., Kaul, S.C., Wadhwa, R., Sundar, D. Computational insights into the potential of withaferin-A, withanone and caffeic acid phenethyl ester for treatment of aberrant-EGFR driven lung cancers. *Biomolecules* 2021, 11: 160. doi:10.3390/biom11020160.

Malik, V., Radhakrishnan, N., Kaul, S.C., Wadhwa, R., Sundar, D. Computational identification of BCR-ABL oncogenic signaling as a candidate target of withaferin A and withanone. *Biomolecules* 2022, 12: 212. doi:10.3390/biom12020212.

Mehta, V., Chander, H., Munshi, A. Mechanisms of anti-tumor activity of Withania somnifera (Ashwagandha). *Nutr Cancer* 2021, 73: 914–926. doi:10.1080/01635581.2020.1778746.

Mirjalili, M.H., Moyano, E., Bonfill, M., Cusido, R.M., Palazon, J. Steroidal lactones from *Withania somnifera*, an ancient plant for novel medicine. *Molecules* 2009, 14: 2373–2393. doi:10.3390/molecules14072373.

Namdeo, A.G., Ingawale, D.K. Ashwagandha: Advances in plant biotechnological approaches for propagation and production of bioactive compounds. *J Ethnopharmacol* 2021, 271: 113709. doi:10.1016/j.jep.2020.113709.

Oh, E., Garg, S., Liu, Y., Afzal, S., Gao, R., Yun, C. O., Kaul, S. C., Wadhwa, R. Identification and functional characterization of anti-metastasis and anti-angiogenic activities of tri-ethylene glycol derivatives. *Front Oncol* 2018, 8: 552. doi:10.3389/fonc.2018.00552.

Priyandoko, D., Ishii, T., Kaul, S.C., Wadhwa, R. Ashwagandha leaf derived withanone protects normal human cells against the toxicity of methoxyacetic acid, a major industrial metabolite. *PLoS One* 2011, 6: e19552. doi:10.1371/journal.pone.0019552.

Sari, A. N., Bhargava, P., Dhanjal, J. K., Putri, J. F., Radhakrishnan, N., Shefrin, S., Ishida, Y., Terao, K., Sundar, D., Kaul, S. C., Wadhwa, R. Combination of withaferin-A and CAPE provides superior anticancer potency: Bioinformatics and experimental evidence to their molecular targets and mechanism of action. *Cancers (Basel)* 2020, 12: 1160. doi:10.3390/cancers12051160.

Sari, A. N., Dhanjal, J. K., Elwakeel, A., Kumar, V., Meidinna, H. N., Zhang, H., Ishida, Y., Terao, K., Sundar, D., Kaul, S. C., Wadhwa R. A low dose combination of withaferin a and caffeic acid phenethyl ester possesses anti-metastatic potential in vitro: Molecular targets and mechanisms. *Cancers (Basel)* 2022, 14: 787. doi:10.3390/cancers14030787.

Shah, N., Kataria, H., Kaul, S.C., Ishii, T., Kaur, G., Wadhwa, R. Effect of the alcoholic extract of Ashwagandha leaves and its components on proliferation, migration, and differentiation of glioblastoma cells: Combinational approach for enhanced differentiation. *Cancer Sci* 2009, 100: 1740–1747. doi:10.1111/j.1349-7006.2009.01236.x.

Shah, N., Singh, R., Sarangi, U., Saxena, N., Chaudhary, A., Kaur, G., Kaul, S.C., Wadhwa, R. Combinations of Ashwagandha leaf extracts protect brain-derived cells against oxidative stress and induce differentiation. *PLoS One* 2015, 10: e0120554. doi:10.1371/journal. pone.0120554.

Shefrin, S., Sari, A.N., Kumar, V., Zhang, H., Meidinna, H.N., Kaul, S.C., Wadhwa, R., Sundar, D. Comparative computational and experimental analyses of some natural small molecules to restore transcriptional activation function of p53 in cancer cells harbouring wild type and p53(Ser46) mutant. *Curr Res Struct Biol* 2022, 4: 320–331. doi:10.1016/j. crstbi.2022.09.002.

Sundar, D., Yu, Y., Katiyar, S.P., Putri, J.F., Dhanjal, J.K., Wang, J., Sari, A.N., Kolettas, E., Kaul, S.C., Wadhwa, R. Wild type p53 function in p53(Y220C) mutant harboring cells by treatment with Ashwagandha derived anticancer withanolides: Bioinformatics and experimental evidence. *J Exp Clin Cancer Res* 2019, 38: 103. doi:10.1186/s13046-019-1099-x.

Straughn, A.R., Kakar, S.S. Withaferin A: A potential therapeutic agent against COVID-19 infection. *J Ovarian Res* 2020, 13: 79. doi:10.1186/s13048-020-00684-x.

Tomita, T., Wadhwa, R., Kaul, S.C., Kurita, R., Kojima, N., Onishi, Y. Withanolide derivative 2,3-dihydro-3beta-methoxy withaferin-A modulates the circadian clock via interaction with RAR-related orphan receptor alpha (RORa). *J Nat Prod* 2021, 84: 1882–1888. doi:10.1021/acs.jnatprod.0c01276.

Vanden Berghe, W., Sabbe, L., Kaileh, M., Haegeman, G., Heyninck, K. Molecular insight in the multifunctional activities of withaferin A. *Biochem Pharmacol* 2012, 84: 1282–1291. doi:10.1016/j.bcp.2012.08.027.

Vaishnavi, K., Saxena, N., Shah, N., Singh, R., Manjunath, K., Uthayakumar, M., Kanaujia, S.P., Kaul, S.C., Sekar, K., Wadhwa, R. Differential activities of the two closely related withanolides, withaferin A and withanone: Bioinformatics and experimental evidences. *PLoS One* 2012, 7: e44419. doi:10.1371/journal.pone.0044419.

Wadhwa, R., Konar, A., Kaul, S.C. Nootropic potential of Ashwagandha leaves: Beyond traditional root extracts. *Neurochem Int* 2016, 95: 109–118. doi:10.1016/j.neuint.2015.09.001.

Wadhwa, R., Yadav, N. S., Katiyar, S. P., Yaguchi, T., Lee, C., Ahn, H., Yun, C.O., Kaul, S. C., Sundar, D. Molecular dynamics simulations and experimental studies reveal differential permeability of withaferin-A and withanone across the model cell membrane. *Sci Rep.* 2021, 11: 2352. doi: 10.1038/s41598-021-81729-z.

Wadhwa, R., Kaul. S. C. Experimental evidence to the untapped potential of Ayurvedic herb, Ashwagandha: Bench-to-bedside. *Intl. J Ayurveda Res* 2023, 4: 15–27. doi:10.4103/ijar.ijar_6_23

Wang, J., Zhang, H., Kaul, A., Li, K., Priyandoko, D., Kaul, S.C., Wadhwa, R. Effect of Ashwagandha withanolides on muscle cell differentiation. *Biomolecules* 2021, 11: 1454. doi:10.3390/biom11101454.

Widodo, N., Kaur, K., Shrestha, B. G., Takagi, Y., Ishii, T., Wadhwa, R., Kaul, S. C. Selective killing of cancer cells by leaf extract of Ashwagandha: Identification of a tumor-inhibitory factor and the first molecular insights to its effect. *Clin Cancer Res* 2007, 13: 2298–2306. doi:10.1158/1078-0432.CCR-06-0948.

Widodo, N., Takagi, Y., Shrestha, B.G., Ishii, T., Kaul, S. C., Wadhwa, R. Selective killing of cancer cells by leaf extract of Ashwagandha: Components, activity and pathway analyses. *Cancer Lett* 2008, 262: 37–47. doi:10.1016/j.canlet.2007.11.037.

Widodo, N., Shah, N., Priyandoko, D., Ishii, T., Kaul, S.C., Wadhwa, R. Deceleration of senescence in normal human fibroblasts by withanone extracted from ashwagandha leaves. *J Gerontol A Biol Sci Med Sci* 2009, 64: 1031–1038. doi:10.1093/gerona/glp088.

Widodo, N., Priyandoko, D., Shah, N., Wadhwa, R., Kaul, S. C. Selective killing of cancer cells by Ashwagandha leaf extract and its component withanone involves ROS signaling. *PLoS One* 2010, 5: e13536. doi:10.1371/journal.pone.0013536.

Yu, Y., Katiyar, S.P., Sundar, D., Kaul, Z., Miyako, E., Zhang, Z., Kaul, S.C., Reddel, R.R., Wadhwa, R. Withaferin-A kills cancer cells with and without telomerase: Chemical, computational and experimental evidences. *Cell Death Dis* 2017, 8: e2755. doi:10.1038/cddis.2017.33.

Yu, Y., Wang, J., Kaul, S. C., Wadhwa, R., Miyako, E. Folic acid receptor-mediated targeting enhances the cytotoxicity, efficacy, and selectivity of *Withania somnifera* leaf extract: In vitro and in vivo evidence. *Front. Oncol.* 2019, 9: 602. doi:10.3389/fonc.2019.00602. eCollection 2019.

Zhang, H., Wang, J., Prakash, J., Zhang, Z., Kaul, S. C., Wadhwa, R. Three-way cell-based screening of antistress compounds: Identification, validation, and relevance to old-age-related pathologies. *J Gerontol A Biol Sci Med Sci.* 2023, 78: 1569–1577. doi:10.1093/gerona/glad103.

Index